Arthroscopic Surgery of the Knee

CURRENT PROBLEMS IN ORTHOPAEDICS

This series of monographs, each written or edited by a distinguished authority, deals with special topics in orthopaedics, particularly those which present major problems in diagnosis and management, and where recent research advances carry important implications for patient care.

Editorial Advisory Board

Already published

Menelaus: The Orthopaedic Management of Spina Bifida Cystica
Sevitt: Bone Repair and Fracture Healing in Man

In preparation

Ling: Complications of Total Hip Replacement
Leffert: The Brachial Plexus
Spjut: Bone Tumors
Turco: Club Foot
Samuelson & Freeman: Surgical Treatment of the Arthritic Ankle and Foot
Catterall: Legg-Calvé-Perthes' Disease
Bauer, Galasko & Weber: Radionuclide Scintigraphy in Orthopaedics

Arthroscopic Surgery of the Knee

David J. Dandy, FRCS

Consultant Orthopaedic Surgeon, Newmarket General Hospital and Addenbrooke's Hospital, Cambridge;
Associate Lecturer, Faculty of Clinical Medicine, University of Cambridge.

FOREWORD BY

R. W. Jackson, MD, MS, FRCS(C)
Associate Professor, Department of Surgery, University of Toronto

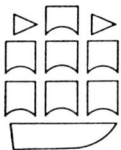

CHURCHILL LIVINGSTONE
EDINBURGH LONDON MELBOURNE AND NEW YORK 1981

CHURCHILL LIVINGSTONE
Medical Division of Longman Group Limited

Distributed in the United States of America by
Churchill Livingstone Inc., 19 West 44th Street, New York,
N.Y. 10036, and by associated companies,
branches and representatives throughout
the world.

First published 1981

ISBN 0 443 02047 7

British Library Cataloguing in Publication Data
Dandy, David J
    Arthroscopic surgery of the knee
    – (Current problems in orthopaedics).
    1. Arthroscopy
    2. Knee – Surgery
    I. Title   II. Series
    617'.582'05   RD561   80–41772

Typeset by CCC, printed and bound in Great Britain by William Clowes
(Beccles) Limited, Beccles and London.

Foreword

The widespread acceptance of arthroscopy as a diagnostic technique, and the development of appropriate arthroscopic surgery instrumentation, has led to the successful fulfillment of the premise, that if you can see pathology, you should be able to deal with it by arthroscopic techniques. In a book that will probably become a classic as the first major text on this subject, David Dandy has beautifully outlined the surgical procedures that are currently possible under arthroscopic control. In his characteristically humorous way, he makes it quite clear that arthroscopic surgery is not only a reality in the present time but also promises exciting prospects for the future. It is obvious that he is describing the new standard of care for many of the pathological lesions that affect the knee, as the morbidity is less and the results are at least equal to (if not better than) open operative procedures. Mr Dandy has produced a timely text, and one that is full of pearls of wisdom. This book represents the beginning of a dramatic new era in knee surgery.

R.W.J., 1981

Preface

The last twenty-five years have seen the development of powerful light sources, glass fibre light guides, optical systems that can transmit a clear image through a telescope less than 2 mm in diameter, and precisely engineered instruments that are both small and strong. These innovations have brought many previously inaccessible anatomical structures within the range of endoscopy, and the knee is one such structure.

Greater experience of arthroscopy, together with the development of suitable operating instruments has made the next step—the performance of intra-articular surgical procedures without arthrotomy—a new and exciting reality. For the patient, the benefits of endoscopic surgery include more accurate diagnosis, more precise surgery, a reduction in surgical trauma and swifter rehabilitation, and for the surgeon a reduction in the demands for hospital beds and physiotherapy.

The skills and techniques needed for this type of surgery are new and must be learnt slowly and painfully through experience. This volume attempts to set down the knowledge gained so far and to provide a foundation on which others may build. The disorders of synovium, ligament, bone, articular cartilage and menisci at present amenable to arthroscopic surgery are set out with details of the technique appropriate to the management of each. Although present experience is meagre and many of the principles put forward will either become obsolete or be proved wrong as surgical techniques become more sophisticated, it is the author's hope that some of the observations made will make it unnecessary for each surgeon to repeat all the mistakes of his predecessors.

In common with other endoscopic procedures such as laparoscopic sterilisation and transurethral resection, there is far more to learning the technique than the purchase of expensive equipment, and no surgeon should consider embarking on arthroscopic surgery of the knee until he is fully confident in his arthroscopic technique. The time taken to reach this goal varies greatly from individual to individual but it is unlikely that sufficient expertise will have been acquired until roughly a hundred arthroscopies have been performed. It is important to concentrate on improving basic arthroscopic skills before attempting the techniques outlined in this book and to avoid the temptation to skimp the groundwork.

The introduction of arthroscopy to an orthopaedic practice that is already working well without it is attended by many practical problems, of which perhaps the greatest is the initial drop in the number of patients treated. Because of this and other difficulties, arthroscopic surgery is unlikely to become routine orthopaedic practice until there is a new generation of orthopaedic surgeons who have grown up with arthroscopy and regard the arthroscope as an instrument just as fundamental to orthopaedic surgery as a bone spike or an osteotome. Until then, and as long as there are self-taught arthroscopists teaching themselves arthroscopic surgery, there will be a need for a basic instructional manual. It is the author's hope that this volume will go some way towards the fulfilment of that need.

Cambridge, 1981   D.J.D.

To Dr R W Jackson

Acknowledgements

I am indebted to many people for their help during the preparation of this book, some for assistance with the development of the surgical techniques described and others for the manuscript itself. For help during the development of the techniques, I am deeply grateful for the skill, patience and forbearance of the operating theatre staff at Newmarket General Hospital, Addenbrooke's Hospital, Cambridge, the Hope Nursing Home and the Evelyn Nursing Home, and in particular, to Staff Nurse M J McGregor at Newmarket; to the entire staff of the Physiotherapy Department and Wards C6 and C7 at Newmarket for their help and constructive criticism of the results of arthroscopic surgery and to Mr M J King and his colleagues at Chas F Thackray Ltd, for assistance in the development of the arthroscope.

For the preparation of the manuscript itself, I am grateful to Mrs M Thorburn for the line diagrams, to the Staff of the Department of Medical Illustration at Addenbrooke's Hospital, Cambridge, and above all, to Mrs S French for her untiring efforts in typing and re-typing the manuscript so frequently.

Finally, I would like to record my thanks for the help and encouragement of my wife Jane, and for the tolerance shown by our children James and Emma, during the entire project which involved a period of intense concentration that they could not share.

Contents

1

The history of arthroscopy and arthroscopic surgery

The history of endoscopy is the history of successive attempts to overcome the frustratingly simple problem of looking down an illuminated tube in such a way that the brilliance of light placed directly at the end of a tube does not enter the observer's eye and make vision beyond impossible. Although the answer to this puzzle has come nearer with the introduction of newer and more efficient sources of light and with successive optical innovations, the perfect solution has yet to be discovered.

The first report of endoscopy in clinical practice was presented by Phillip Bozzini to the Academy of Medicine in Vienna in 1806. In Bozzini's instrument, the 'lichtleiter', light from a beeswax candle passed down a polished silver tube which also served as a speculum (Fig. 1.1). This instrument was first used for examination of the nasopharynx but could also be used to examine the anal canal, rectum, vagina, bladder, urethra, and the interior of bone affected by osteomyelitis. The use of the instrument was painful, the illumination poor, and the field of vision small (Bush et al 1974). Bozzini's audience in Vienna was unreceptive; his paper was greeted with derision and his instrument considered to be of no clinical importance—a reaction which is not unknown after the announcement of more recent advances in endoscopy. Bozzini returned from Vienna to his practice in Frankfurt, where he died three years later at the age of thirty six.

Pierre Ségalas presented an instrument of similar design to the Academie des Sciences in 1826, thereby initiating an acrimonious dispute with Herteloupe who claimed that Ségalas had plagiarised his own idea, which used lampyrids (glow-worms) as a light source. Presumably the glow-worm must have emitted a

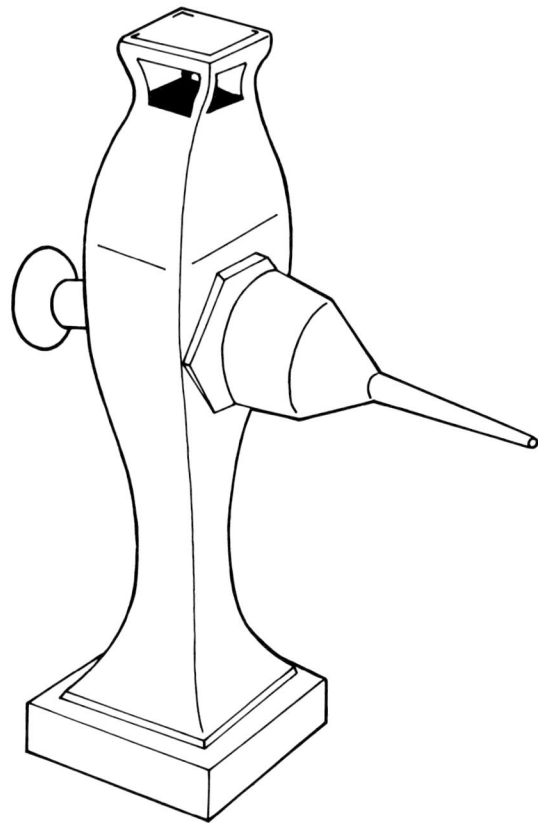

Fig. 1.1 The Bozzini endoscope. This instrument was covered with Morocco leather and the light source was a beeswax candle

constant light rather than an intermittent flash, and the female of the species *lampyris noctiluca*, which is wingless and measures 18 mm in length and 5 mm in diameter, was probably used (Foster, W A 1979). Little more was heard of endoscopy until 1853 when Desormeaux introduced an endoscope in which the light source was a spirit lamp that burned a mixture

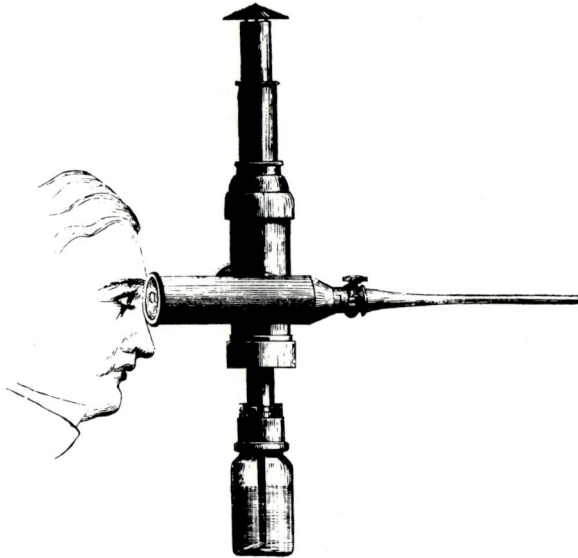

Fig. 1.2 The Desormeaux endoscope in use

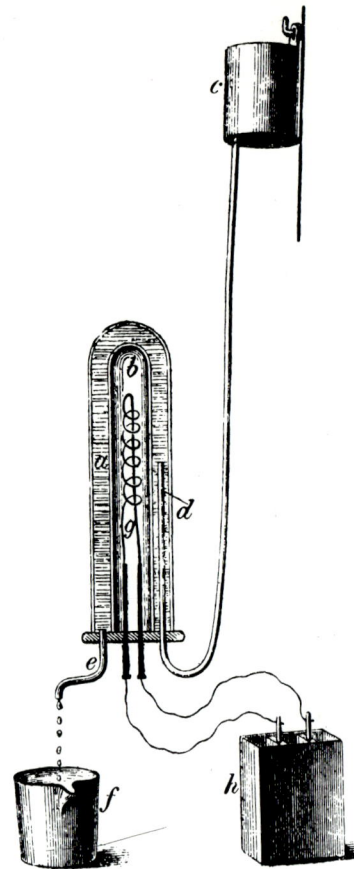

Fig. 1.3 Bruck's lamp (from Fenwick, E H, 1889)

of alcohol and turpentine called 'gazogene' (Fig. 1.2). The optical system included polished silver tubes, mirrors, and lenses. The operation must have been a trial for patient, surgeon and assistants alike. It is easy to imagine a darkened room illuminated only by the lamp of the endoscope, which probably emitted as much heat as light, the smell of burning turpentine mixed perhaps with that of hot paint on a new instrument, and the apprehension of the unanaesthetised but stoical Gallic patient as the proboscis of this terrifying contraption entered his urethra.

Cumbersome though the Desormeaux cystoscope may have been, it survived its critics and was improved by others, among them F R Cruise of Dublin, who in 1865 increased the brilliance of the flame by using a mixture of petrol and camphor and made handling easier by the addition of a mahogany case to protect the surgeon's hands from the heat of the lamp (Murphy 1972).

Other attempts to improve the light source included a burning magnesium filament introduced by J Andrew in 1867, and Bruck's diaphanoscope. Bruck's innovation is worthy of mention not only because it was the forerunner of the electric lamp, but because it demonstrated the determination and enterprise of the endoscopic pioneers. Julius Bruck was a dentist of Breslau who in 1867 developed a platinium filament that could be raised to white heat by electricity from a battery and cooled by a glass jacket though which water flowed (Fig. 1.3). Straying beyond the normal confines of dentistry, Bruck placed this crude electric

light source in his patient's rectum so that the interior of the bladder could be observed through a straight speculum passed along the urethra. A gynaecologist colleague of Bruck found that if the lamp was placed in the vagina, he could make out the shape of the uterus and ovaries 'in a thin woman in a darkened room' (Wallace 1978).

Max Nitze (1848–1906) developed Bruck's lamp further, and in 1877 fitted a heated platinum filament shielded by a window of rock crystal and cooled by a continuous flow of water to the end of an endoscope so that the light source itself was introduced into the bladder (Fenwick 1889). This instrument was improved with the help of Leiter, an instrument maker of Vienna, and in 1879 the Nitze-Leiter cystoscope was produced (Fig. 1.4). The lighting and cooling systems of this instrument fell short of perfection, and the invention was ridiculed as a 'fire and water contraption'.

In 1878 Swan, an Englishman, preceded Edison by several months in producing an incandescent lamp which was first fitted to an endoscope by David

Arthroscopy

The first endoscopes were used for viewing the bladder, rectum or vagina and it was not until 1918 that Professor K Takagi of Tokyo examined the interior of the knee. The instrument used was a cystoscope, but Takagi quickly developed an instrument specifically designed for the knee. This instrument, which he called an 'arthroscope', was 7.3 mm in diameter and had no lens system. The principal use of the instrument in Japan in those days lay in the management of tuberculosis of the knee which, through ankylosis, made squatting and kneeling impossible and led to serious social and physical incapacity. The Takagi instruments later included a lens system and evolved rapidly, permitting black and white photography of the interior of the knee in 1932 (Takagi 1933), followed by ciné photography and colour photography in 1936 (Takagi 1939).

Independently of Takagi, Eugen Bircher of Aarau in Switzerland reported in 1921 the results of twenty 'arthro-endoscopic' examinations of the knee using the Jacobeaus laparo-thoracoscope, first distending the knee with oxygen or nitrogen by means of an artificial pneumothorax apparatus. The work of Takagi and Bircher stimulated much interest and it was not long before arthroscopy reached the English speaking world. In 1925, Philip H Kreuscher presented details of the use of the arthroscope in the early diagnosis of meniscal lesions to the Illinois Medical Society. The study of arthroscopy continued and advanced at the Hospital for Joint Diseases in New York, where Dr Michael Burman used an instrument with an outside diameter of 4 mm, designed by R Wappler, to examine the elbow, ankle and shoulder as well as the knee (Burman 1933; Burman, Finkelstein and Mayer 1934; Burman and Mayer 1936; Mayer and Burman 1939).

In Europe, the work of Bircher sometimes met the same crushing scepticism that had greeted the work of Bozzini and Nitze in the previous century. In 1937, Hustinx, who had no experience of the instrument or its use, wrote 'But what to think of the gonoscope which Bircher advocated at the Accident Congress held in Amsterdam in 1925? How can anyone venture to introduce a luminous object into the knee joint in an effort to look between the articular surfaces, which cannot be separated? Even at arthrotomy it is impossible to see the posterior horn of the meniscus if the knee joint is not sufficiently open. How then

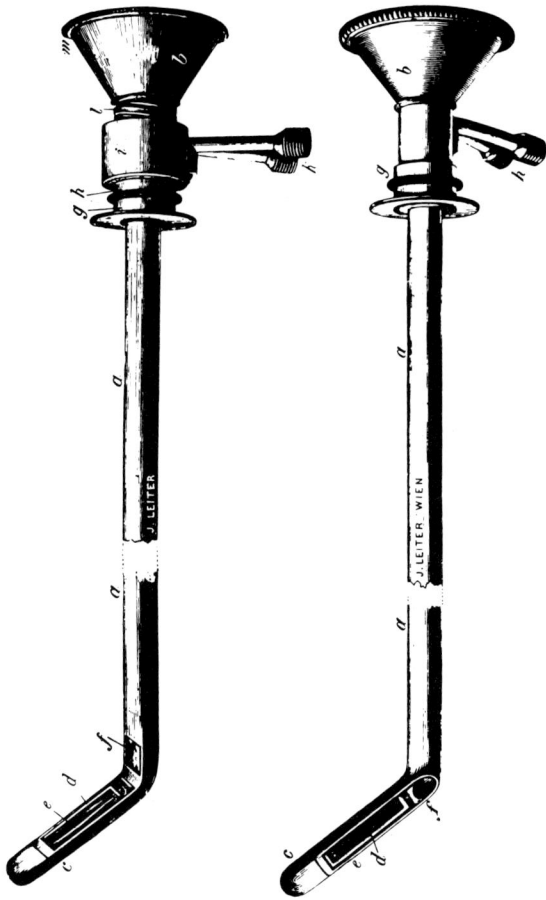

Fig. 1.4 The Nitze-Leiter cytoscope (1879). The electric filament (e) covered by a rock crystal window (d) illuminated the bladder, which could be observed through the lens (f) (from Fenwick E H 1889)

Newman of Glasgow in 1883. Leiter subsequently used the same lamp in 1886, and was followed by Nitze in 1887 to produce a cystoscope remarkably similar in appearance to those in use today. Later advances in optical design included the Amici prism which for the first time produced an upright instead of an inverted image, and refinements in lens manufacture and design improved the quality of the image still futher.

Optical design continues to progress and two recent innovations, both introduced by Professor H H Hopkins of Reading University, have done much to improve the reliability and versatility of endoscopy. These two innovations are the rod lens system, which makes possible the construction of smaller telescopes that produce a better image with less light loss than was previously possible, and the glass fibre light guide now used in all modern endoscopes.

could one expect to see it in a closed joint? This is quite impossible. Moreover, this procedure is more dangerous than an exploratory arthrotomy.' (Eikelaar 1975.)

Despite such opposition, the work continued and arthroscopy was on the point of becoming an established technique when all work in Japan, North America and Europe was brought to an abrupt halt by the Second World War. When hostilities were ended, several years passed before arthroscopy again progressed. In 1957 Takagi's successor, Dr Masaki Watanabe, published his Atlas of Arthroscopy which included water colour illustrations and was followed in 1969 by a second edition that included endoscopic photographs. Of Watanabe's many contributions to arthroscopy, perhaps the greatest was the number 21 arthroscope (Fig. 1.5), which was introduced in 1960, and became the instrument of choice for arthroscopists around the world for a decade.

In Europe and North America, interest in arthroscopy had been virtually extinguished by the Second World War. Dr I Macnab of Toronto used a paediatric cystoscope to examine the interior of a knee in 1963 (Jackson 1979), but general interest in arthroscopy was not rekindled until Dr R W Jackson returned to Toronto in December of 1964 after working with Dr Watanabe. The teaching of Dr Jackson has since influenced many surgeons in America, Europe and Australasia, and has done more than anything else to establish arthroscopy as a routine clinical procedure in the English speaking world. The first North-American course in arthroscopy was held in Philadelphia in 1972 where, in 1975, arthroscopy finally became established with the inauguration of the International Arthroscopy Association under the

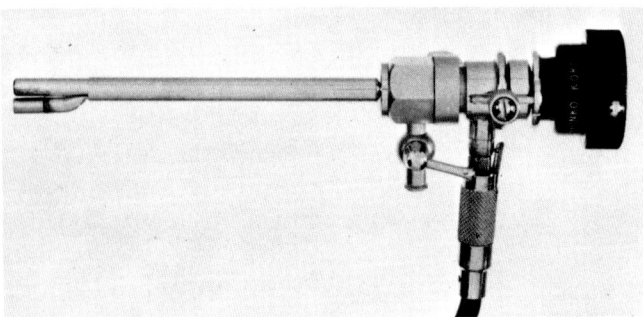

Fig. 1.5 The Watanabe 21 arthroscope. This instrument, with an off-set tungsten light bulb mounted on a separate light carrier, laid the foundations of modern arthroscopy (photograph by courtesy of Colonel J Carson, USAF)

Presidency of Professor Masaki Watanabe. The first European course was held in 1976, at Nijmegen under the direction of Professor T Van Rens, and courses have since been held in Scandinavia in 1977 and England in 1979.

Arthroscopic surgery of the knee

It has proved impossible to discover who was the first to perform arthroscopic surgery of the knee but the idea appears to have been published first by E S Geist in 1926 when he wrote in a 'preliminary report' of the possibility of synovial biopsy through the arthroscope; 'We ought not only to be able to see through this tube inserted into the joint, but, like the genito-urinary surgeon, we ought to be able with suitable instruments to procure from the joint the necessary pathological material for microscopic study.

'As I conceive it, the performance of arthroscopy in the living ought not to be more distressing to the patient than a simple aspiration, provided local anaesthesia is employed.

'Further communications will follow.'

Sadly, there seems to have been no further communication until Lipson, Clemmons and Frymoyer described the successful results of arthroscopic synovial biopsy in 1967. The procedure has since become popular among rheumatologists, often conducted under local anaesthesia just as Geist envisaged.

Dr M Watanabe became the first to perform an arthroscopic meniscectomy when he removed a posterior flap tear of the medial meniscus in 1962 (Carson, R W 1979; O'Connor, R L 1979; Ikeuchi, H 1979. Dr R W Jackson removed two loose bodies from the knee in 1966 (Jackson, 1979) and a bucket handle fragment of meniscus in 1970, since when arthroscopic surgery has been developed by Dr R L O'Connor and others. Surprisingly, there do not seem to have been any reports of the clinical results of arthroscopic surgery until 1978 (Dandy, D J 1978).

Arthroscopic surgery is now following arthroscopy on the road to becoming an accepted technique, with courses held in Maine in 1978 and during 1979 in Finland, Denver, and Hawaii, where over three hundred surgeons attended a course organised by Dr R L O'Connor. The speed and enthusiasm with which arthroscopic surgery has been accepted by orthopaedic surgeons around the world is an indication of its remarkable success, but should also sound a note of warning. After such an explosion of enthusiasm there must follow a trough of disappointment and disillusion with many reports of failures and complications. Those who take up arthroscopic surgery should not allow themselves to be depressed by such reverses any more than they should be influenced by the present elation but should instead persevere until arthroscopic surgery finds its true place in the therapeutic arsenal of the orthopaedic surgeon.

REFERENCES

Bircher E 1921 Die arthroendoskopie. Zentralbl Chir 48: 1460–1461.

Bozzini P 1806 Lichtleiter, eine Erfindung zur Anschauung innerer Theile und Krankheiten nebst der Abbildung, in Hufeland C W (ed), Journal der practischen Arzneykunde und Wundarzneykunst Berlin 24: 107–124.

Burman M S 1931 Arthroscopy or direct visualization of joints. An experimental cadaver study. Journal of Bone and Joint Surgery 13: 669–695.

Burman M S, Mayer L 1936 Arthroscopic examination of the knee joint. Archives of Surgery 32: 846.

Burman M S, Finkelstein H, Mayer L 1934 Arthroscopy of the knee joint. Journal of Bone and Joint Surgery 16: 255–268.

Bruck J 1867 Das Urethroskop . . . Durch Galvansches Gluhlicht, Breslau.

Bush R B, Leonhardt H, Bush I M, Landes R R 1974 Dr Bozzini's Lichtleiter. A translation of his original article (1806). Urology, 3, 119–123.

Carson R W 1979 Arthroscopic Meniscectomy. Orthopaedic Clinics of North America 10: 619–627.

Dandy D J 1978 Early Results of Closed Partial Meniscectomy. British Medical Journal 1: 1099–1100.

Desormeaux A J 1853 De L'Endoscope. Bull Acad Med Academie des Sciences 1855.

Eijkelaar H R 1975 Arthroscopy of the knee—Thesis for a doctorate in orthopaedic surgery at the University of Groningen, The Netherlands. Royal United Printers Hoitsema B V

Fenwick E H 1889 The Electric Illumination of the Bladder and Urethra. J and A Churchill, London.

Foster W A 1979 Personal communication.

Geist E S 1926 Arthroscopy: preliminary report. Journal-Lancet Minneapolis 46: 306–307.

Herteloupe C L S 1827 La Lithotritie. Academie des Sciences, Paris.

Hustinx E J H 1937 Letsels van de menisci van het kniegewricht. Nederlands Tijdschrift voor Geneeskunde 81 Nr: 12 biz: 1218.

Ikeuchi H 1979 Meniscus Surgery using the Watanabe Arthroscope. Orthopaedic Clinics of North-America 10: 629–64.

Jackson R W 1979 Personal communication.

Kreuscher P 1925 Semilunar cartilage disease, a plea for early recognition by means of the arthroscope and early treatment of this condition. Illinois Medical Journal 47: 290–292.

Lipson R L, Clemmons J J, Frymoyer J W 1967 Arthroscopy: Experience with percutaneous biopsy of intraarticular structures under direct vision. Arthritis Rheum 10: 294.

Mayer L, Burman M S 1939 Arthroscopy in the diagnosis of meniscal lesions of the knee joint. American Journal of Surgery 43: 501.

Murphy L J T 1972 History of Urology. Springfield, Illinois.

O'Connor R L 1979 Personal communication.

Takagi K 1933 Practical experience using Takagi's arthroscope. Journal of the Japanese Orthopaedic Association 8: 132.

Takagi K 1939 The arthroscope. Journal of the Japanese Orthopaedic Association 14: 359–441.

Wallace D M 1978 in 'Handbook of Urological Endoscopy' Gow J G and Hopkins H H Churchill-Livingstone, Edinburgh.

Watanabe M, Takeda S 1960 The number 21 arthroscope. Journal of the Japanese Orthopaedic Association 34: 1041.

Watanabe M, Takeda S, Ikeuchi H 1957 Atlas of Arthroscopy. Igaku Shoin Ltd, Tokyo.

Watanabe M, Takeda S, Ikeuchi H 1969 Atlas of Arthroscopy 2nd ed. Igaku Shoin Ltd, Tokyo.

2

Diagnostic arthroscopy

It cannot be emphasised too strongly that arthroscopic surgery should only be attempted by surgeons who have total confidence in their arthroscopic technique. To identify an abnormality which can subsequently be examined more thoroughly at arthrotomy is easy, but to identify the pathology and anatomy of a lesion precisely enough to be able to insert the appropriate operating instruments at the correct site demands confidence of a different order. Perhaps the greatest danger of arthroscopic surgery is the possibility of inexperienced enthusiasts believing that the purchase of a set of instruments will enable them to perform the operations about to be described before they have mastered the basic techniques, and visions of the havoc that could be wrought by such individuals is the source of great anxiety to those who advocate arthroscopic surgery.

The diagnostic technique required for arthroscopic surgery differs from routine arthroscopy only in the stress laid upon the need for precise identification of pathological anatomy and in the need to become familiar with more than one approach, but it must be remembered that there is much more to a full arthroscopic examination of the knee than simply looking down the arthroscope and admiring the view as if it were a series of still photographs. The movement of the intra-articular structures can be assessed as the knee is flexed and extended as rotary or lateral stresses are applied. Percutaneous needles can be used to inspect the under-surface of the meniscus or to check the stability of its rim and most important of all, probing hooks passed through a second channel can be used to manipulate suspicious structures or to assess the stability of the posterior third of the meniscus if its integrity is in doubt. To omit these additional techniques and rely only on the view down the arthroscope is to conduct a partial arthroscopy, with results that can only be disappointing (Gillies and Seligson 1979).

Indications for arthroscopy

Although the indications for arthroscopy are now generally established and will be well known to any surgeon with enough experience of arthroscopy to contemplate arthroscopic surgery, they bear repetition if only to reiterate that arthroscopy is neither a substitute for clinical acumen nor a short cut to the correct diagnosis.

Arthroscopy is indicated before any arthrotomy for an internal derangement of the knee, in the assessment of complex knee problems such as ligament injuries or persistent symptoms following meniscectomy, in the investigation of supposed hysterics or malingerers and in the diagnosis of acute injuries followed by haemarthrosis for which no cause is apparent. The patient's account of his symptoms and their onset can provide as much information as clinical examination, radiography and arthroscopy combined and arthroscopy does not supplant the clinical history as the single most useful weapon in the investigation of any knee disorder. The findings of arthroscopy cannot be considered in isolation and are useful only if they can be correlated with the patient's symptoms and the findings of clinical and radiological examination.

Equipment

When selecting an arthroscope, it is advisable to choose a model which does not have a bridge. A bridge was necessary in the original paediatric cystoscopes from which most arthroscopes have evolved because of the need for ureteric catheterisation and biopsy of the bladder wall, but a bridge is not necessary for diagnostic arthroscopy and can easily be omitted accidently when the instrument is assembled in the knee. If the bridge is not inserted, several centimetres of unprotected telescope will protrude from the sheath of the instrument, and there is a real risk of the telescope breaking at the end of the sheath. There are now numerous cases of arthroscopes breaking in this way with unfortunate consequences for both the patient and the surgeon. The most effective insurance against this mishap is to purchase an instrument which does not include a removable bridge.

The straightahead 0° telescope is recommended for the novice arthroscopist because its field of vision lies directly in front of the telescope and the direction in which the arthroscope is pointing can be used as a reliable guide to orientation (Fig. 2.1). Although the 30° telescope makes it possible to see areas inaccessible to the 0° telescope, anatomical landmarks within the

joint must be used for navigation and a little experience is required before these landmarks can be recognised easily, but any surgeon considering arthroscopic surgery should already be thoroughly familiar with arthroscopic anatomy and be able to use the 30° arthroscope with confidence. The work-horse of arthroscopic surgery is the 5 mm rod lens arthroscope with a 30° fore-oblique lens, but different brands of arthroscopes are now so similar that it is difficult to choose between them and most surgeons will prefer to continue using their diagnostic instrument for arthroscopic surgery.

A 70° telescope is very helpful in the detailed assessment of the postero-medial and postero-lateral compartments and is strongly recommended as a useful addition to the basic set of instruments (Fig. 2.2). The small diameter arthroscope (Fig. 2.3), if used in conjunction with the multiple puncture technique popularised by Johnson (Johnson 1977, Johnson and Becker 1976) is very satisfactory for diagnostic arthroscopy and can well be used for out-patient diagnosis under local anaesthesia, but the advantages of this instrument disappear if the surgeon then proceeds to use a large instrument for the operative stage of the procedure. Without detracting from the virtues of Johnson's technique as a purely diagnostic procedure under local anaesthesia, the larger diagnostic instruments with an outside diameter of 5 mm offer a clearer view of wider area and are the instruments of choice if arthroscopy is a preliminary to arthroscopic surgery.

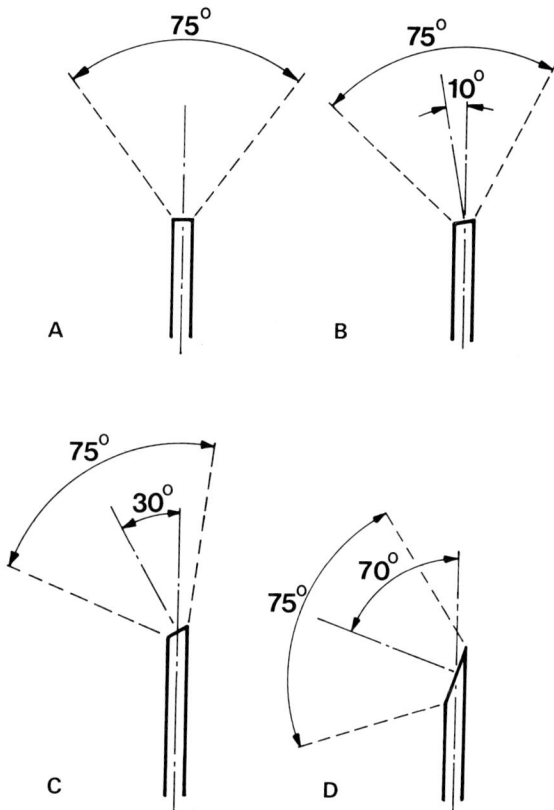

Fig. 2.1 The direction of vision of the arthroscope. (a) straightahead arthroscope; (b) 10° fore-oblique (sometimes referred to as 170°); (c) 30° fore-oblique; (d) 70° fore-oblique

Preparation

Anaesthesia

General anaesthesia has many advantages for both the surgeon and the patient. The injured knee, particularly that with a locked meniscus, is frequently painful and the forceful manipulation of the joint necessary to identify the exact anatomy of some lesions is an unnecessary discomfort for the patient and a hindrance to the surgeon. General anaesthesia also avoids the need for repeated infiltration of the skin when it becomes necessary to insert the arthroscope at a second site, or to probe the meniscus with the hook or percutaneous needles. Moreover, many arthroscope procedures are best done under tourniquet control and the use of a tourniquet on the unanaesthetised patient for more than a few minutes is unkind.

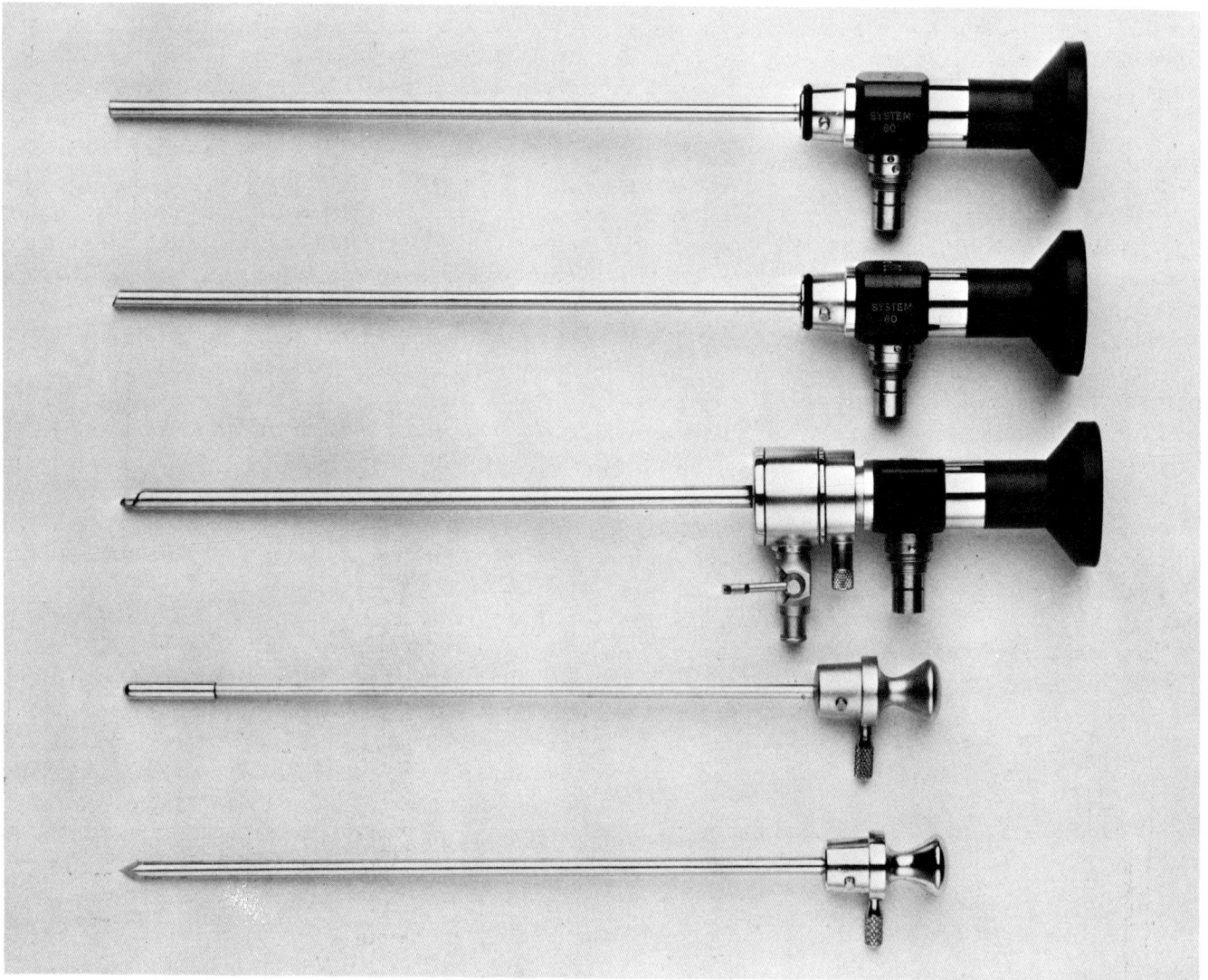

Fig. 2.2 A set of arthroscopes. From above downwards; 0° telescope, 30° telescope, 70° telescope in sheath, blunt obturator and sharp trocar

Perhaps the greatest advantage of general anaesthesia is that it renders the patient oblivious to events in the operating theatre. It is by no means unusual for a planned operation to change imperceptibly into an *ad hoc* procedure requiring the sterilisation of additional instruments and the rejection of those already prepared. On these occasions, the confidence of the patient and the credibility of the surgeon are more likely to survive the operation intact if the patient is asleep.

Although general anaesthesia is preferred, local anaesthesia is quite feasible both for diagnostic and operative arthroscopy provided that the surgeon is experienced and confident in his technique. The skin and subcutaneous tissues should be infiltrated with bupivacaine 0.5 per cent containing added adrenaline

along the medial and lateral joint lines and the site of insertion of the irrigation needle. Bupivacaine can also be added to the irrigation fluid (McGinty and Matza 1978). The use of adrenaline minimises any haemorrhage that may occur from the site of insertion of the arthroscope, and efficient irrigation is usually sufficient to ensure a fairly clear field of view without the use of a tourniquet.

Tourniquet

The use of a tourniquet has the disadvantage that the subtleties of synovial vascularity are lost, but it also has the single great advantage that bleeding can be effectively controlled. If arthroscopic surgery is planned, the appearance of the synovium is likely to

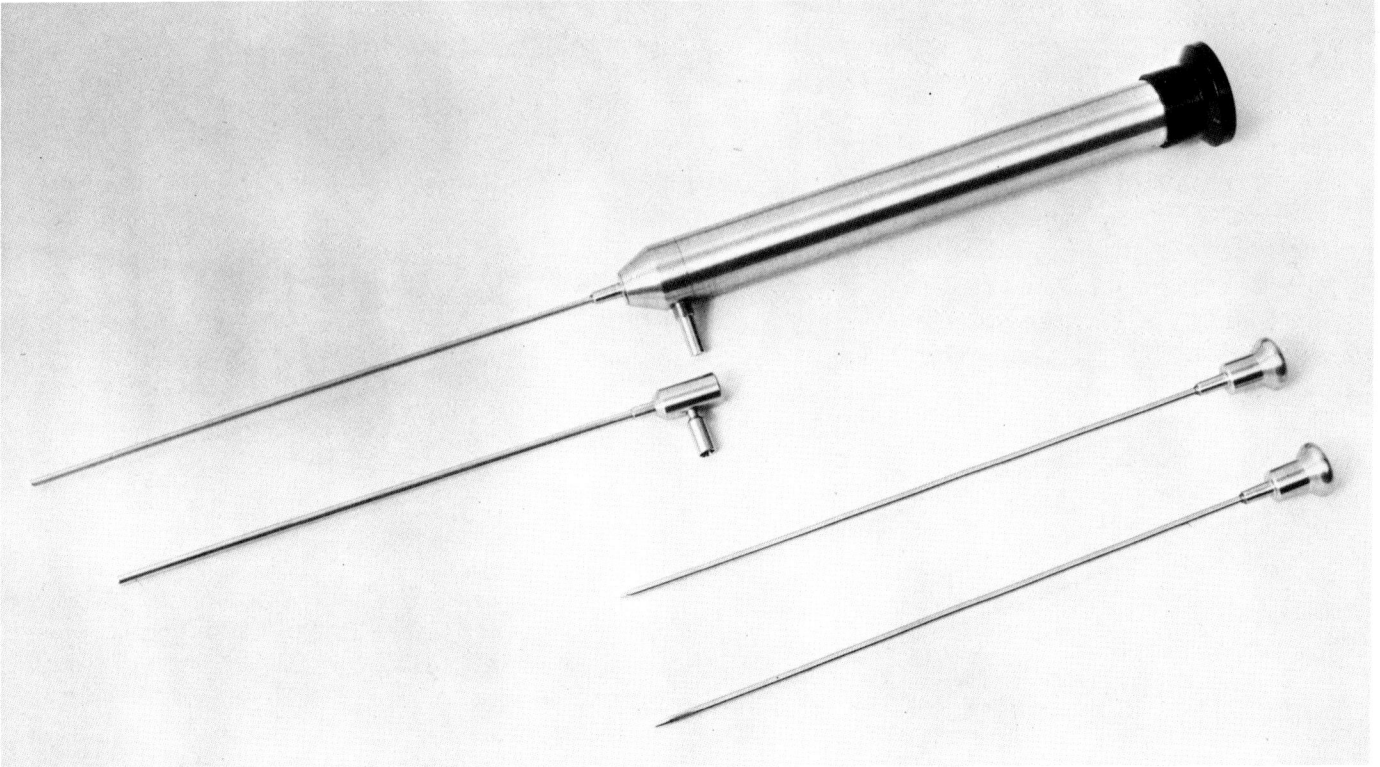

Fig. 2.3 The Dyonics Needlescope. From above downwards; Needlescope, sheath, sharp trocar, and blunt obturator

be of less importance than the control of haemorrhage and it is therefore prudent to apply an uninflated pneumatic tourniquet to the thigh in all cases. If there is a possibility that the arthroscopy will be followed by an arthroscopic meniscectomy or other procedure, the leg may be elevated and the tourniquet inflated before the towels are applied, but this step can be deferred until the arthroscopy is completed if the appearance of the synovium is of particular importance. In the author's practice, the patient's leg is now elevated and the tourniquet inflated as a routine, omitted only if specifically indicated. Exsanguination is unnecessary and blanches the synovium to such an extent that even the identification of the menisco-synovial junction may be difficult.

If inflation of the tourniquet becomes necessary to control haemorrhage on the increasingly rare occasions when it is not inflated before the limb is draped, the arthroscope should be withdrawn and the leg elevated for at least one minute before inflation. If this precaution is omitted or the tourniquet inflated with the knee flexed over the edge of the table, severe venous congestion of the leg may ensue with an increased risk of venous thrombosis. At the end of the procedure, the tourniquet should be released and the joint irrigated thoroughly until the effluent fluid is clean.

Irrigation

Continuous irrigation of the joint is helpful during any arthroscopic procedure and the system used for the preliminary diagnostic arthroscopy can be used without modification, the irrigation fluid entering the sheath of the arthroscope and leaving through a needle in the suprapatellar pouch. Number 18 gauge needles are often used in spinal anaesthesia and are therefore readily available and, with the infusion bag or bottle one metre above the knee, ensure a steady flow of fluid through the joint without allowing the synovial cavity to collapse.

The needle is best used without a tube attached. Although the drainage of the fluid down a plastic tube and into a bucket can reduce the spillage of irrigation fluid, the drainage tube is an unnecessary addition to the complex array of tubes and light cables that already attend arthroscopy, and the presence of such a tube makes it difficult to know whether the needle has become blocked. The weight of the tube itself is also a disadvantage, not only because it may tilt the needle so that its tip comes to lie against the synovium and become blocked, but also because its weight may pull the needle out of the joint altogether.

The irrigation fluid of choice is normal saline suitable for intravenous injection or irrigation, but sterile water can also be used. Although the use of sterile water might appear undesirable on the grounds that it could enter the circulation, especially if there is a tear of the posterior joint capsule which could allow the fluid to escape into the calf, it has the advantage that any stray red cells are promptly haemolysed. Despite the potential hazards, sterile water has been used routinely in some centres, sometimes under pressure, without ill-effect or cause for regret.

Examination under anaesthesia

Examination under anaesthesia plays an important part in investigation of the knee, particularly if a ligament injury is suspected, and should always precede arthroscopy (Fig. 2.4). The patient should be fully relaxed before the examination is conducted. A quick tussle with the leg in the anaesthetic room immediately after induction is of no value, but time spent on a careful examination for the anterior or posterior draw sign and the pivot shift sign of MacIntosh is time well invested.

Skin preparation and draping

The leg should be shaved before operation to avoid the risk of hairs being driven into the joint on the tip of the arthroscopic trocar, and the skin prepared as if an arthrotomy were to be performed. Arthroscopy has no place as an unsterile 'office procedure' and should only be performed in a fully-equipped operating theatre. Because it is virtually impossible to avoid the surgeon's mask, eyelashes or hood touching either his gloves or the patient's leg during the examination, the procedure ceases to be truly sterile as soon as the eye is brought to the eyepiece. Some degree of sterility can be maintained by insisting that all instruments should be handled by the handle or eyepiece only, and that *nobody* should touch the barrel of the arthroscope or any instrument that might enter the joint.

The leg should be draped in such a way that the leg and knee can be manipulated freely without risk of

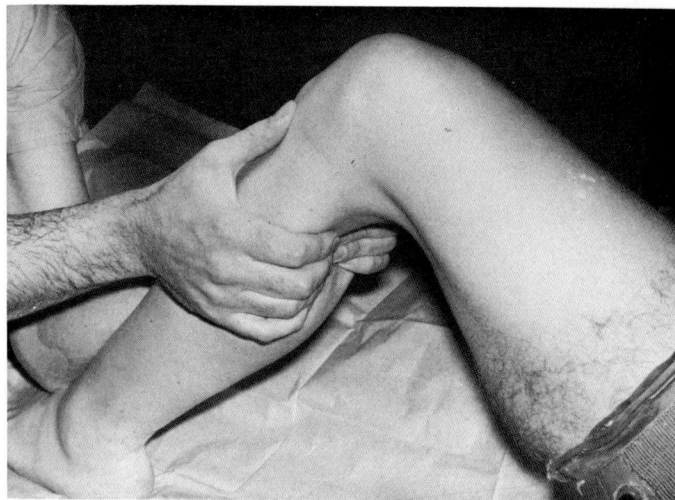

Fig. 2.4 Examination of the knee under general anaesthesia

the towels, irrigating tube or light cable falling to the floor. The towels around the calf and the foot should be applied firmly so that they do not come adrift when the knee is manipulated, and should not be so bulky or irregular that the surgeon's mask or cap is likely to brush against them any more than can be avoided. Although it is true that there are many ways in which the towels can be arranged to satisfy these simple requirements and that any surgeon attempting arthroscopic surgery will already have discovered a method that suits his own arthroscopic technique, it may still be helpful to describe one routine that has proved effective.

The patient is anaesthetised in the anaesthetic room, and when fully relaxed is placed on the operating table and the knee carefully examined. The leg is then elevated, a pneumatic tourniquet applied and inflated by a technician or assistant while the surgeon scrubs, and a diathermy plate applied in the usual way in case an arthrotomy is necessary. With the leg still elevated, a waterproof sheet is placed across the table and under the leg, and the skin prepared from the middle of the calf to the level of the tourniquet with an appropriate antiseptic solution, such as 0.5 per cent chlorhexidine in 70 per cent alcohol (Fig. 2.5). The first sterile waterproof sheet is then replaced with a second and covered with a large sterile linen sheet. A small square towel is then folded into a triangle, wrapped around the thigh at the junction of its lower and middle thirds, and secured with two towel clips which do not enter the skin. The leg is then lowered into a second small towel which is laid under the leg and the towel wrapped carefully

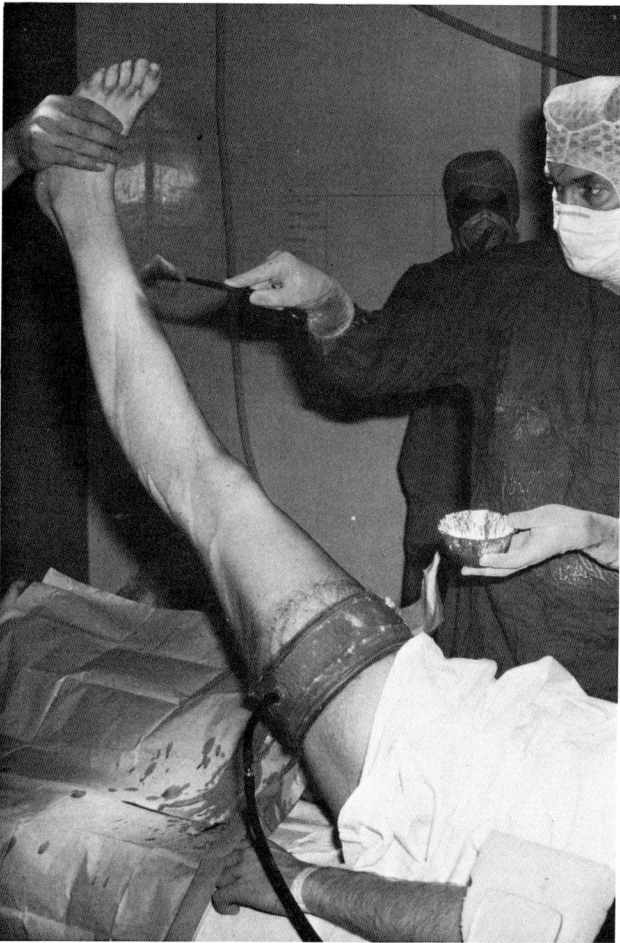

Fig. 2.5 Preparation of the leg with antiseptic solution after application of a tourniquet

and neatly around the calf and foot, to be secured throughout its length with a 10 cm (4″) wide cotton bandage tied in such a way that the knot lies on the inner side of the calf or ankle. This part of the draping must be done neatly and correctly. If the towel is crumpled untidily around the calf or secured loosely with some feeble material such as tubular gauze, the drapes will inevitably slide down to the ankle at the most inconvenient and difficult stage of the procedure.

A large abdominal sheet with a central hole is then passed over the leg and secured with a towel clip. The sterile light cable and sterile intravenous infusion is laid over the abdomen, held with a clip in a fold of towel at the level of the groin, and covered with another sheet. A good length of cable and tube should be left free to allow easy manipulation of the arthroscope without tension on either cable or tube (Fig. 2.6).

Positioning of the infusion set, light source, instrument trolley and assistant is important (Fig. 2.7). The assistant should stand next to the surgeon, towards the patient's head. The drip set and light source should be at the patient's head, preferably on the side away from the surgeon with the instrument trolley on the opposite side of the surgeon, and not at the foot of the table where the surgeon is certain to back into it during the procedure.

Distension of the joint

A little irrigation fluid is then run into a sterile container, drawn up into a 20 of 50 ml syringe, and the knee inflated by injecting the saline into the suprapatellar pouch through a No. 18 gauge needle. To inject the saline into the sub-synovial layers instead of into the synovial cavity is surprisingly easy. Examination of the joint is certain to be difficult when this occurs and the intra-articular manipulation of operating instruments may be rendered completely impossible but attention to the following points should help to avoid this mishap. Firstly, care should be taken

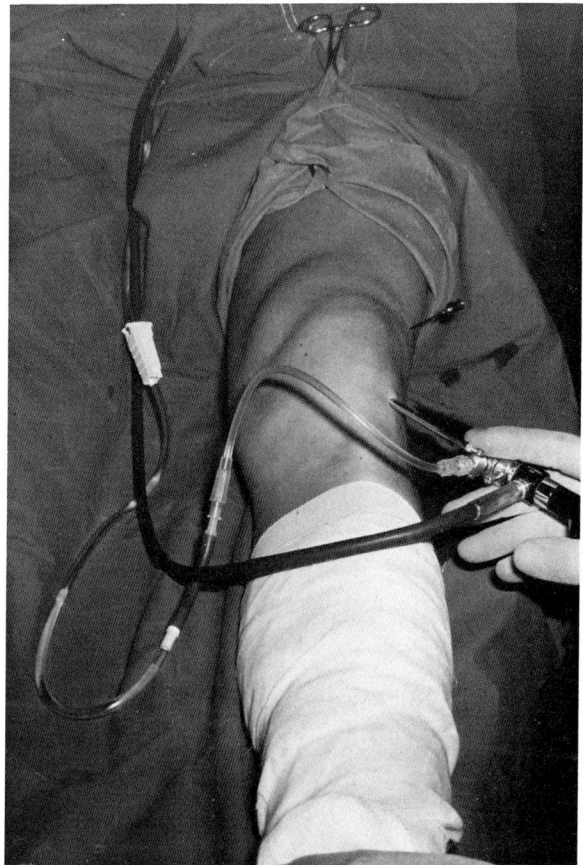

Fig. 2.6 The draped leg with the irrigation tube, light cable, drainage needle and arthroscope in position

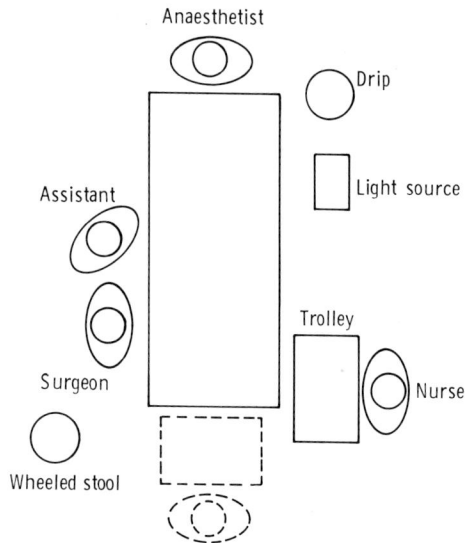

Fig. 2.7 Theatre layout. For arthroscopic surgery the instrument trolley can be brought to the position indicated by a broken line at the end of the operating table

that the needle is inserted at the supero-lateral angle of the patella and the under-surface of the patella felt with the side of the needle before any saline is injected. A few millilitres of saline may then be injected into the joint and the medial side of the knee watched carefully to be certain that the fluid is seen running down into the medial gutter (Fig. 2.8). If in doubt, the syringe can be detached to see if any fluid runs

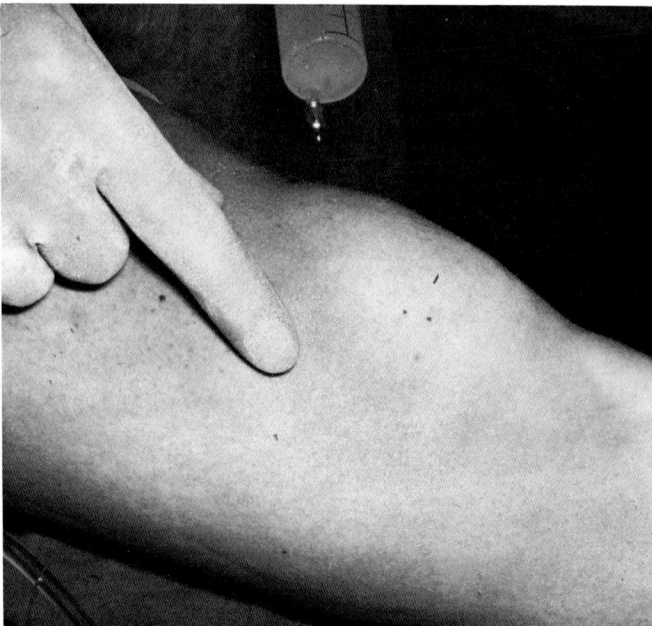

Fig. 2.8 Irrigation fluid running down in the medial gutter, confirming that the needle tip is correctly placed in the synovial cavity

back along the needle. When it is certain that the needle is well in the joint, the needle should be held still and a further 20–50 millilitres of fluid injected to lift the patella off the underlying femur. If there is any real doubt that the needle lies in the joint, it is wiser to desist and insert the instrument carefully into a dry joint rather than risk the disaster of obliterating the joint cavity with a soggy mass of oedematous sub-synovial tissue. With the joint inflated, the stylet should be placed in the needle to prevent the joint emptying and preparations made for insertion of the arthroscope.

Routine examination from the antero-lateral approach

Of the many possible points of insertion of the arthroscope (Whipple and Bassett 1978), the antero-lateral insertion as described by Dr R W Jackson and based on the technique of Dr M Watanabe (Jackson and Abe 1972; Jackson and Dandy 1976), is the most useful for routine initial examination of the knee. It must be remembered that the antero-lateral approach was originally developed for use with the old Watanabe 21 instrument, which had a tungsten bulb at its tip that made it impossible to pass the instrument along the narrow tunnels which have become passable with the advent of smaller instruments and glass fibre light guides. Although it is essential for the surgeon attempting arthroscopic surgery to become familiar with several insertions, an established routine approach for the initial examination is important and the antero-lateral approach serves this purpose well.

Insertion of the arthroscope

The point of insertion for the antero-lateral approach lies 2 mm above the anterior horn of the lateral meniscus and as close to the patellar tendon as possible (Fig. 2.9). This point can best be identified by flexing the knee to 90° and pushing the thumbnail into the small depression just lateral to the patellar tendon. A 5 mm incision extending down through the joint capsule is then made with a small No. 15 blade immediately above the thumbnail (Fig. 2.10). With a sharp trocar locked into the arthroscope sheath, and the forefinger laid along the barrel of the instrument to prevent unexpected plunging of the tip, the trocar is directed upwards, medially and backwards towards the intercondylar notch, and driven through the

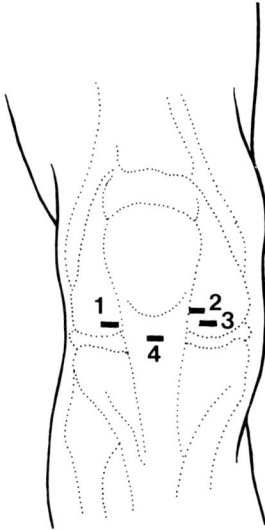

Fig. 2.9 Site of insertion of the arthroscope 1. Antero-lateral approach 2. Antero-medial approach 3. Lower and more medial point of insertion for approaching the posterior horn with operating instruments 4. Central approach

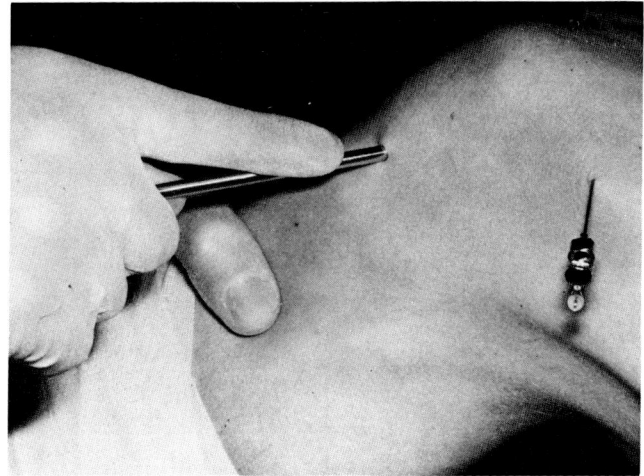

Fig. 2.11 Inserting the arthroscopic trocar

capsule with a gentle screwing movement (Fig. 2.11). A slight pop is usually felt as the joint capsule is penetrated and the joint entered.

The next stage of the procedure is to lift the patella on the tip of the sheath and pass the instrument into the suprapatellar pouch as the knee is straightened. Some surgeons prefer to replace the sharp trocar with a blunt obturator before straightening the knee, but the trocar will not damage the surface providing that care is taken and the joint is full of saline. It is

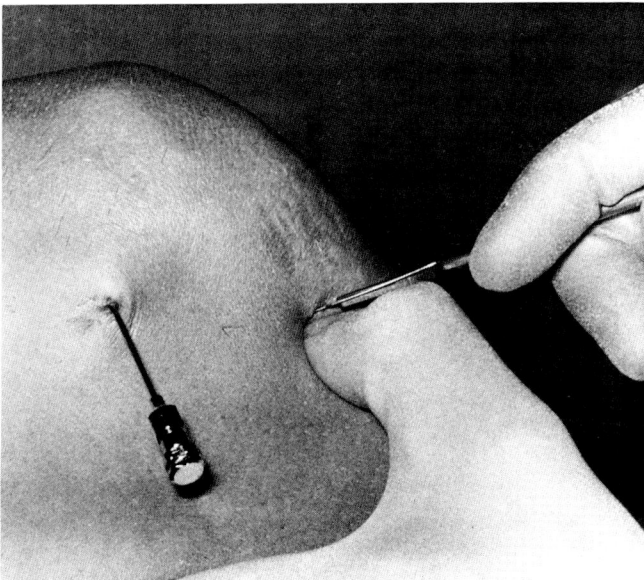

Fig. 2.10 Incising the skin before inserting the arthroscope from the antero-lateral approach

important to make certain that no 'assistant' is holding the patient's leg during this manoeuvre for any interference with the smooth movement of the instrument can lead to unnecessary trauma to the articular cartilage and even damage to the instrument.

Assembly of the instrument

With the sheath in the suprapatellar pouch, the trocar can be withdrawn and the joint washings examined. Yellow or bloodstained fluid may be taken as evidence of an intra-articular disorder and the presence of flecks or flakes of articular cartilage in the washings indicate either generalised osteoarthrosis or synovial chondromatosis. The joint is then irrigated thoroughly until completely clear fluid is obtained, or visibility within the joint will be poor.

The instrument should then be assembled by insertion of the telescope and attachment of the light cable and irrigation tube. If the arthroscope includes a bridge, care must be taken to ensure that it is inserted correctly and locked into position. As mentioned already, failure to insert the bridge leaves several centimetres of telescope unprotected by the sheath, with the very real risk that the telescope can be bent or broken inside the knee. Although many excellent arthroscopes include a bridge as evidence of their distant origins as paediatric cystoscopes, instruments specifically designed for arthroscopy omit this dangerous design feature.

Suprapatellar pouch

Because of the irregular shape of the lower end of the femur and the convolutions of the synovial cavity that

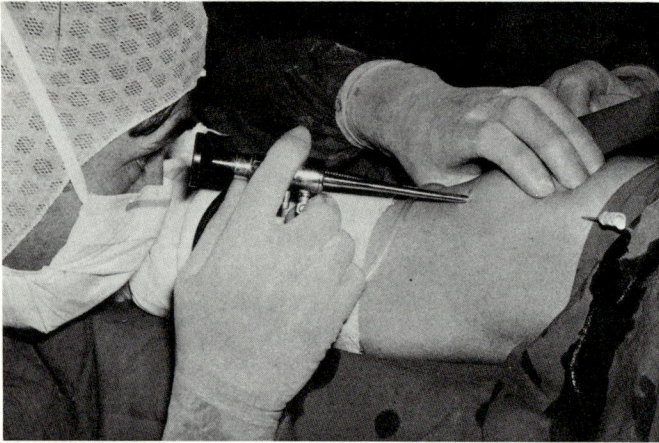

Fig. 2.12 Examining the under-surface of the patella

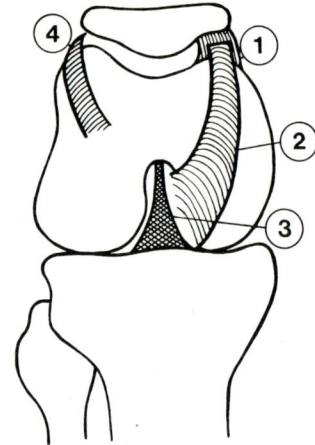

Fig. 2.13 The synovial folds in the knee 1. Medial suprapatellar plica 2. Medial synovial shelf 3. Ligamentum mucosum 4. Lateral synovial shelf

surround it, thorough examination of the knee involves manipulation of the leg around the end of the arthroscope as well as manipulation of the arthroscope inside the joint. These manoeuvres are made unnecessarily difficult if the surgeon immobilises himself by sitting down during the procedure. Apart from the disadvantage of immobility, the initial arthroscopy should take only a few minutes and there is no time for sitting.

The examination begins in the suprapatellar pouch (Fig. 2.12), which is most easily examined with the table raised so that the patient's knee is at the level of the surgeon's umbilicus. The telescope is placed first at the apex of the pouch, with the line of vision directed medially. The first structure to be identified

should be the medial suprapatellar plica (alias the plica synovialis suprapatellaris and plica medialis suprapatellaris) (Fig. 2.13) which lies on the medial side of the joint and may divide the pouch into two almost separate compartments (Fig. 2.14). Attention to this area is important because the medial suprapatellar plica can conceal much interesting pathology, and afford a hiding place for loose bodies (Fig. 5.1). It may also be noted that when the knee is affected by generalised synovitis, particularly that associated with osteoarthritis, the changes of synovitis in the synovium hidden behind the plica are less marked than in the rest of the joint.

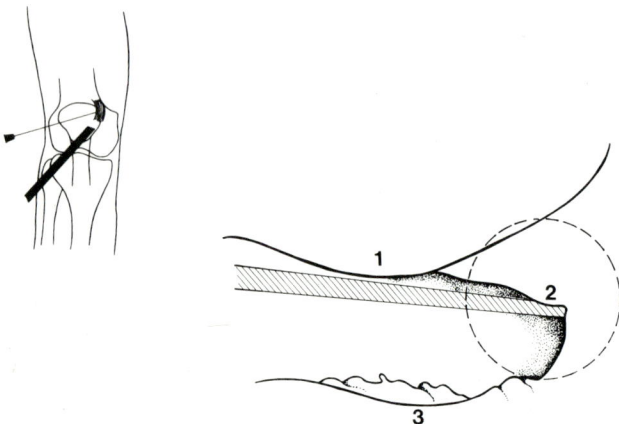

Fig. 2.14 The medial suprapatellar plica (1) manipulated with the irrigation needle (2) patella (3) femur
N.B. All arthroscopic photographs represent the right knee

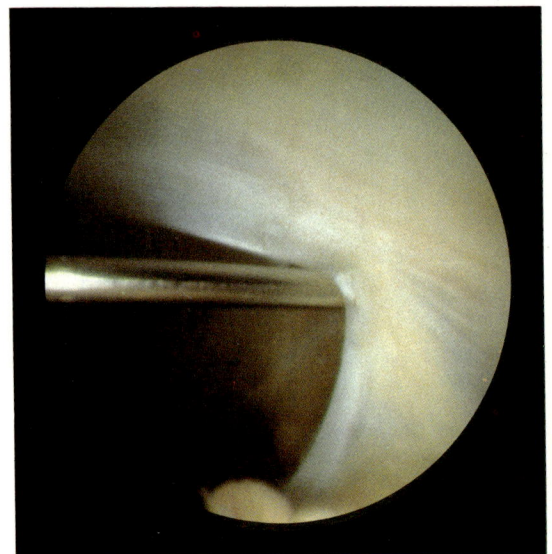

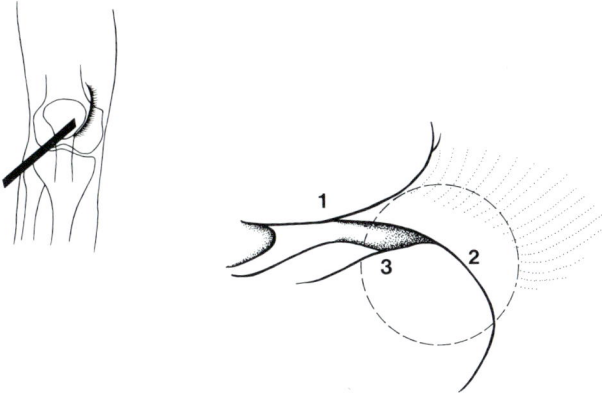

Fig. 2.15 The medial synovial shelf (2) (1) patella (3) medial femoral condyle

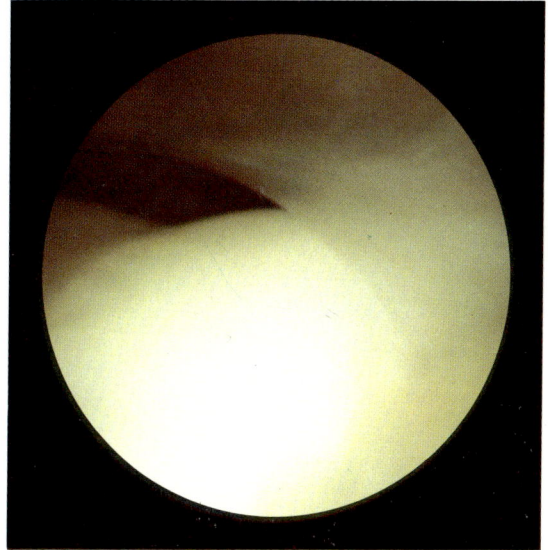

The telescope should then be withdrawn slightly, and the appearance of the synovium in the rest of the suprapatellar pouch examined. If the synovium is inflamed, special note should be made of the shape of the villi, which will appear fatter and rounder in acute synovitis than in a chronic synovitis in which they are finer and filiform.

Patello-femoral joint

The surface of the patella is examined next by withdrawing the arthroscope slightly and rotating the barrel so that the line of vision is directed upwards. The articular cartilage can then be scanned from side to side for degenerative changes or evidence of osteochondral fractures and any suspicious areas probed with the irrigation needle (Fig. 5.13). By moving the patella across the tip of the telescope, the whole surface of the patella may be examined with the 30° telescope, although the 70° telescope is very occasionally needed to examine the upper pole of the patella and the under-surface of the patellar tendon. The relationship of the patella to its groove is important, and can be assessed most easily from the lateral gutter, as described on p. 19.

The direction of vision should next be aimed medially and slightly upwards to search for the medial synovial shelf (alias the plica synovialis medio patel-laris, plica alaris elongata, Iino's band, Aoki's ledge, meniscus of the patella, medial patellar plica) which runs in the coronal plane and ends in the fat pad below the inferior pole of the patella. The shelf, which was first reported by Iino (1939) and has since been described by Patel (1978) is visible as a white crescent (Fig. 2.15), but may be thickened and inflamed if the rest of the joint is affected by synovitis or if there has been localised trauma to the shelf itself. The white crescentic appearance of a thickened shelf is similar to that of the meniscus so that it is sometimes aptly referred to as the 'meniscus of the patella'.

A similar fold of synovium may also be seen on the lateral side of the patella, but the lateral 'shelf' is neither as clean nor as sharp as its medial counterpart (Fig. 2.16). Special attention should be paid to both these folds if there is parapatellar tenderness, or if the patient has symptoms referrable to the patello-femoral joint.

Medial compartment

The medial compartment is the next area to be examined and can be entered by turning the telescope downwards to identify the edge of the medial femoral condyle and rolling the tip of the arthroscope around the condyle as the knee is flexed over the edge of the table to bring the medial meniscus into view. The menisco-synovial junction should then be identified and inspected for peripheral meniscal tears and localised synovitis before proceeding to a thorough examination of the meniscus itself. The edge of the

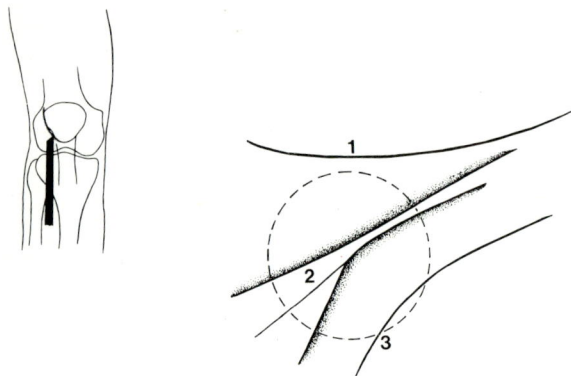

Fig. 2.16 The lateral synovial shelf (2) (1) patella (3) lateral femoral condyle

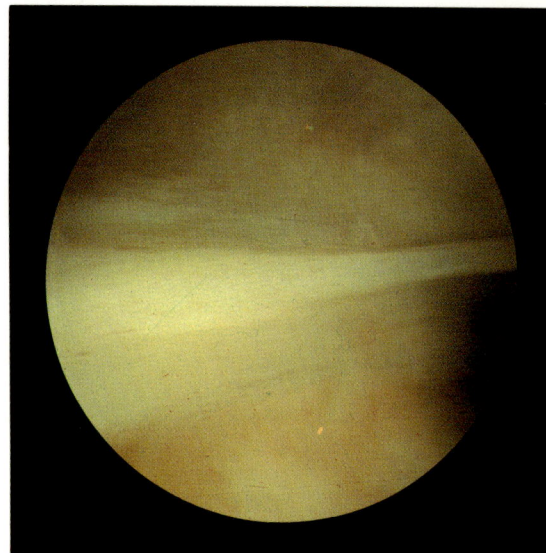

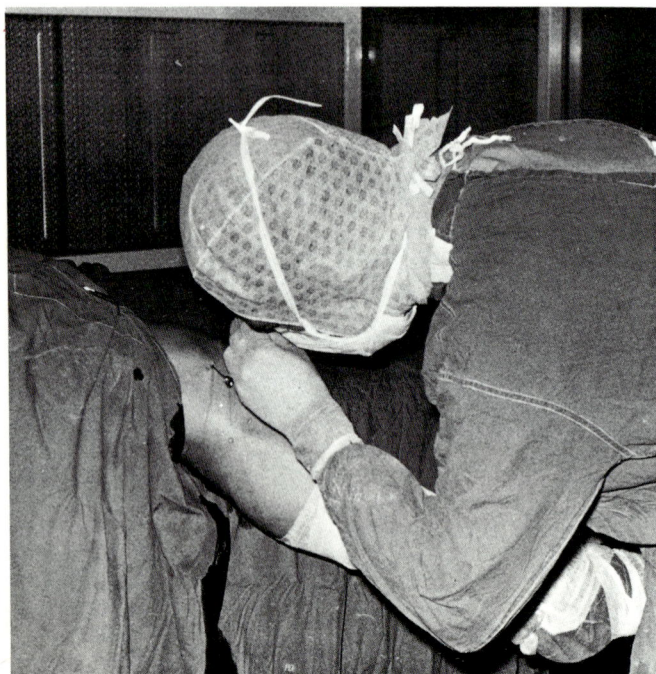

Fig. 2.17 Applying a valgus stress in external rotation to open up the medial compartment

medial meniscus can almost always be seen throughout its length by applying a firm valgus and external rotation strain with the knee in 30° of flexion (Fig. 2.17), a manoeuvre which sometimes displaces concealed meniscal flaps into the joint space (Figs. 6.29, 6.30). More information about the posterior horn will be obtained during the examination of the postero-

medial compartment but there are many times when routine visual inspection does not provide complete information about the meniscus and the use of percutaneous probing needles, the probing hook, or a postero-medial insertion of the arthroscope become necessary.

Before leaving the medial compartment, the articular surface of the femoral condyle should be examined for irregularities and for the 'impingement lesion' that is often seen at the point of contact of the medial femoral condyle and the anterior horn of the medial meniscus in full extension (Figs. 2.18, 2.19). This lesion, which is not uncommon and may be asymptomatic, appears as an area of heaped up tissue immediately above a slight depression at the base of which there may be irregular articular cartilage. The lesion frequently comes into contact with the medial synovial shelf during flexion and may well be one cause of symptoms in the synovial shelf syndrome. Whatever its significance, the presence of this lesion and its relationship to the synovial shelf should be established and recorded.

The intercondylar notch

Examination of the intercondylar notch may be made difficult by the presence of synovitis, folds of synovium, meniscal fragments or osteophytes. The anterior cruciate ligament is a convenient landmark which can be identified by slipping the arthroscope laterally out

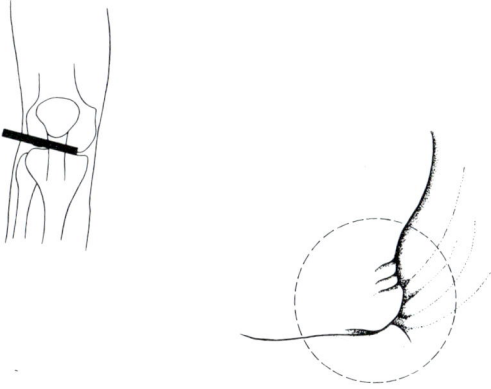

Fig. 2.18 The 'impingement lesion', consisting of an area of heaped up and softened articular cartilage at the point of impingement of the medial femoral condyle and the anterior horn of the medial meniscus

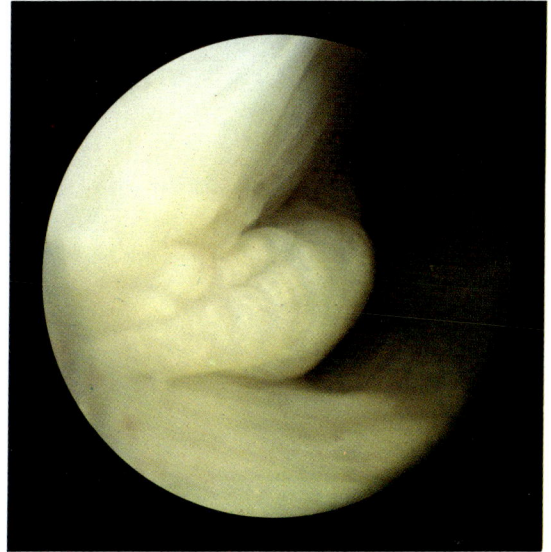

of the medial compartment while withdrawing it slightly. Care must be taken not to withdraw the arthroscope so far that its tip enters the sub-synovial fat-pad because if this is done the saline issuing from the tip of the sheath will quickly distend the sub-synovial tissues and make thorough examination impossible. Once the anterior cruciate has been identified, its fibres should be followed upwards and backwards to the centre of the joint to be certain that it is intact, taking care not to confuse folds of

synovium with the ligament itself. Structures in this area are close to both the lens and the light source and thus appear unnaturally white and excessively magnified. Difficulty in passing the arthroscope across the notch may be caused by the ligamentum mucosum (alias the plica synovialis infrapatellaris, inferior patellar plica, or inferior synovial fold) which is the anatomical vestige of the septum which once divided the knee into separate medial and lateral compartments. The ligamentum mucosum is variable in extent

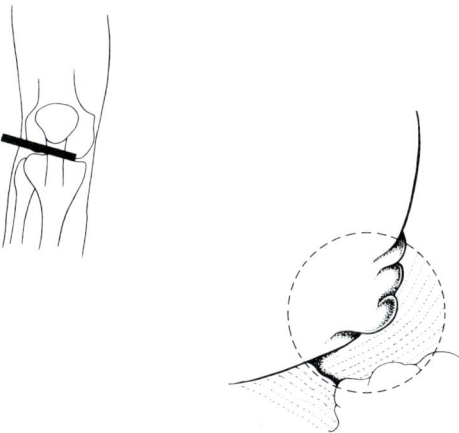

Fig. 2.19 The 'impingement lesion' seen with the knee slightly flexed and the lesion raised above the anterior horn of the medial meniscus

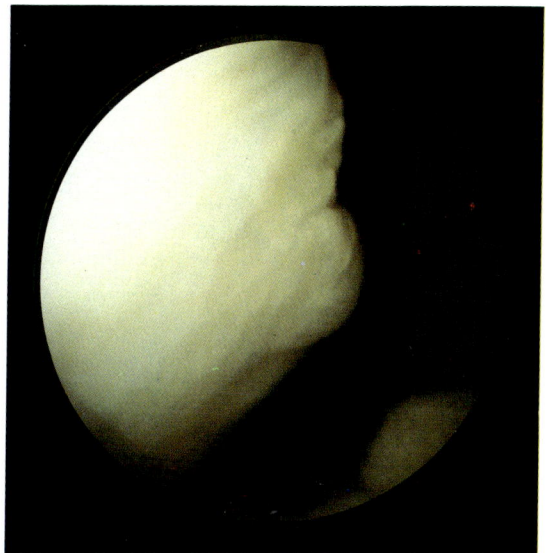

and thickness but can almost always be negotiated by keeping the tip of the arthroscope as close to the anterior cruciate ligament as possible so that it passes beneath the obstruction.

Before leaving the notch, the arthroscope may be turned upwards to inspect the small fat-pad overlying the attachment of the posterior cruciate ligament to the medial femoral condyle, and medially towards the classical site of osteochondritis dissecans.

The lateral compartment

The lateral compartment is entered by passing the arthroscope laterally while opening the joint space with a varus strain in approximately 30° of flexion. This strain can most conveniently be applied by applying the surgeon's thigh to the outer side of the patient's ankle using the edge of the table as a fulcrum (Fig. 2.20), and will bring the meniscal edge into view throughout its length in almost every patient.

This method of examining the lateral compartment of the knee differs slightly from that described by R W Jackson (Jackson and Dandy 1976), in which the patient's foot is put on the operating table in such a way that the knee falls outwards, with the hip abducted and flexed (Fig. 2.21). Although a good view

of the lateral compartment can be obtained with the knee in this position, manipulation of instruments within the joint is difficult, the position of the leg is harder to control precisely, and loose bodies tend to gravitate to the recess beneath the posterior horn of the lateral meniscus or the postero-lateral compartment, from which retrieval may be difficult (Fig. 2.22). If there is a real possibility that a loose body is lying under the posterior horn of the lateral meniscus, the arthroscope should be passed beneath the meniscus and the recess examined before leaving the lateral compartment.

When the entire meniscus has been inspected, the articular surface of the femoral condyle should be examined by scanning its surface with the tip of the telescope as the knee is flexed and extended, making a note of any craters or irregularities. The telescope is then guided into the lateral gutter and the popliteus tendon brought in view (Fig. 2.23). Although pathology in this area is unusual, loose bodies may be found lurking around the popliteus tendon and localised synovitis around the popliteus tendon is sometimes seen. Before leaving the lateral gutter, the arthroscope should be turned upwards to assess the relationship of the lateral edge of the patella and the underlying femur. If the patella overhangs the edge of the femur

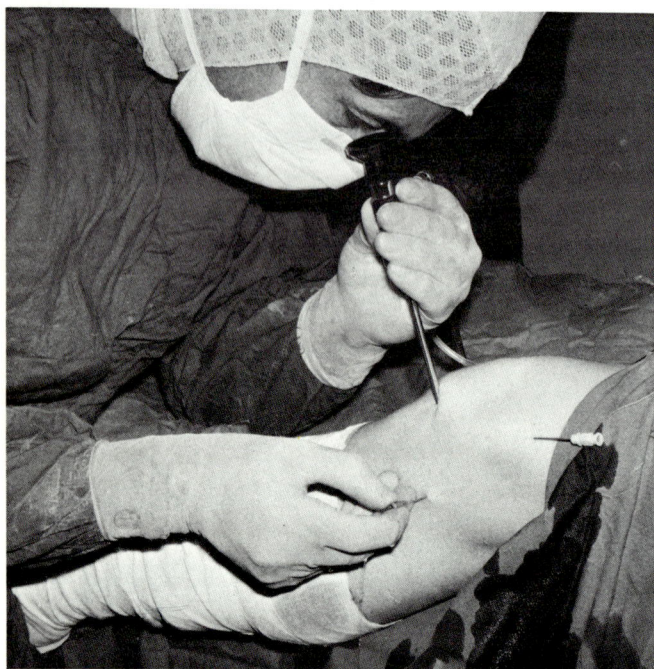

Fig. 2.20 Applying a varus stress to the knee using the edge of the table as a fulcrum, while manipulating the lateral meniscus with a percutaneous needle

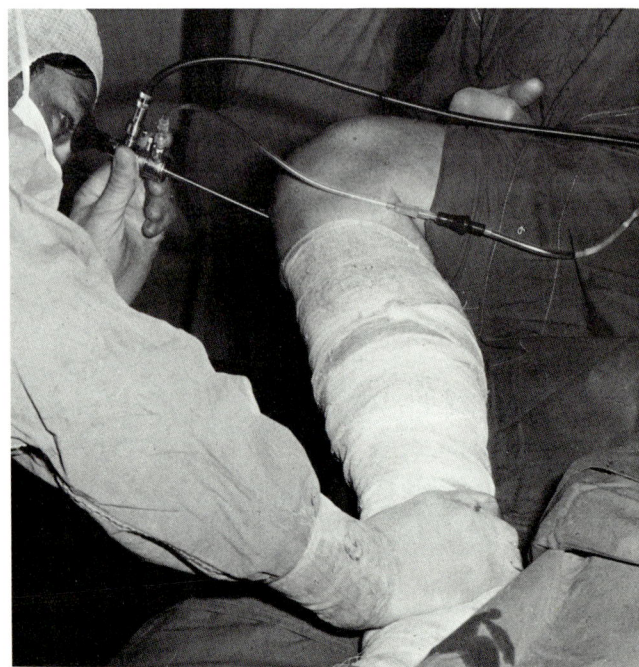

Fig. 2.21 Examining the lateral compartment with the patient's foot on the table. The most dependent part of the joint is the postero-lateral corner

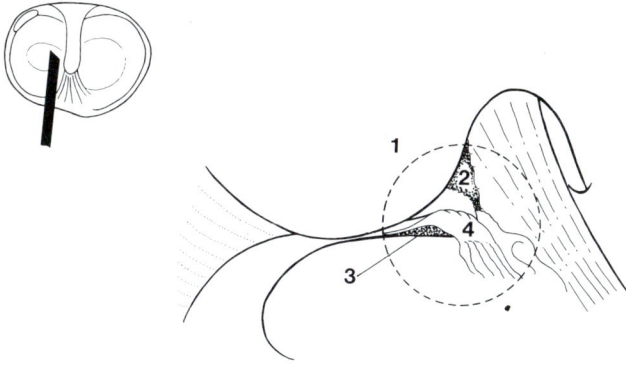

Fig. 2.22 The posterior horn of the meniscus seen from the antero-lateral approach. The opening (2) below the lateral femoral condyle (1) and above the lateral meniscus (4) leads to the postero-lateral compartment. The opening (3) beneath the lateral meniscus leads to a recess in which loose bodies and foreign bodies may become lodged

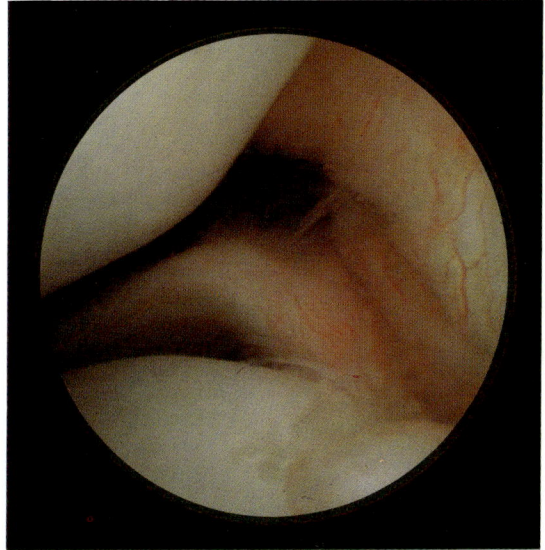

by one third of its width or more (Fig. 4.11), abnormal lateral tracking of the patella is probably present and lateral release of the extensor mechanism may be indicated if the patient's symptoms are arising from the patello-femoral joint.

Great difficulty is occasionally encountered in passing the telescope across to the lateral compartment from the intercondylar notch even when there is no large ligamentum mucosum, and should alert the surgeon to the possibility that there may be a bucket handle fragment of meniscus or a loose body lodged in the notch itself. If the telescope cannot be brought into the lateral compartment through the intercondylar notch, it should be returned to the suprapatellar pouch and passed down to the lateral compartment via the lateral gutter, taking care to manipulate the telescope gently past any synovial folds that obstruct its passage.

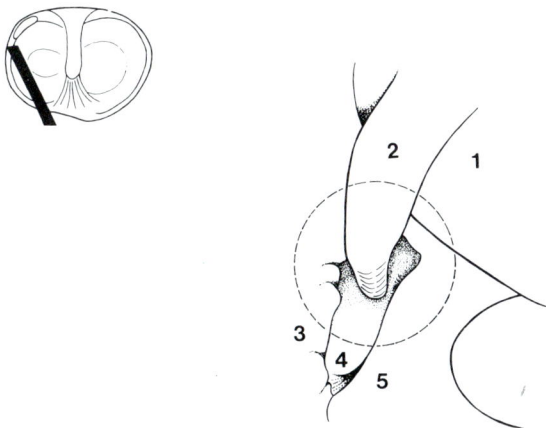

Fig. 2.23 The popliteus tendon (2) entering its tunnel (4) with the knee in slight flexion; (1) femur (3) synovium of lateral gutter (5) lateral meniscus

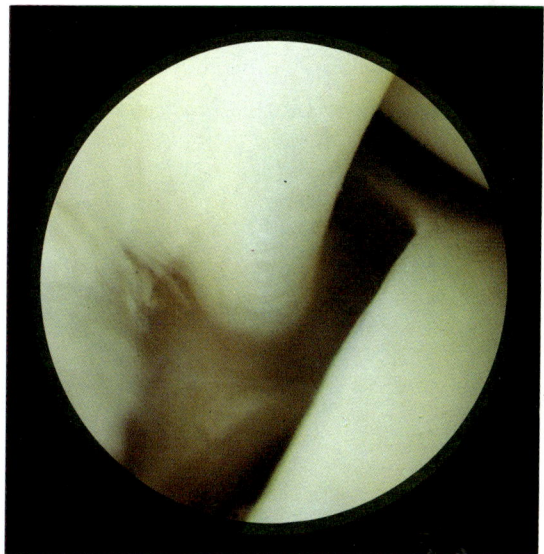

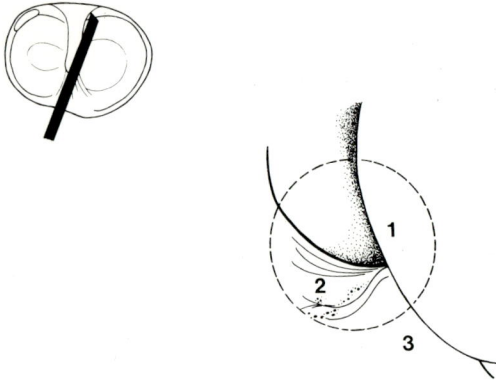

Fig. 2.24 Postero-medial compartment of the knee from the antero-lateral approach. The speckled appearance of the synovium (2) is sometimes seen and is probably a normal variant; (1) medial femoral condyle (3) medial meniscus

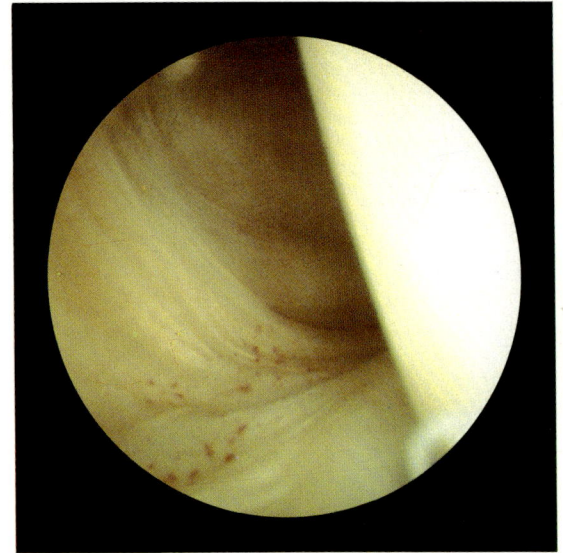

Postero-medial compartment

The postero-medial compartment of the knee is entered by passing the telescope between the medial femoral condyle and the anterior cruciate ligament. This manoeuvre can be achieved from the antero-lateral approach in most knees if the leg is held in external rotation and the knee flexed to approximately 30°, provided that there are no osteophytes or folds of inflamed synovium in the notch to obstruct the passage of the arthroscope (Fig. 2.24). The posterior

attachment of the medial meniscus can be seen clearly as the telescope enters the compartment. When the compartment has been entered and examined with the 30° telescope, the back of the medial meniscus can be examined in more detail with the 70° telescope. Special attention should also be paid to the lateral wall of the compartment where a ruptured posterior cruciate ligament may be seen (Fig. 2.25) and to the floor where loose bodies and other debris often settle (Fig. 6.25).

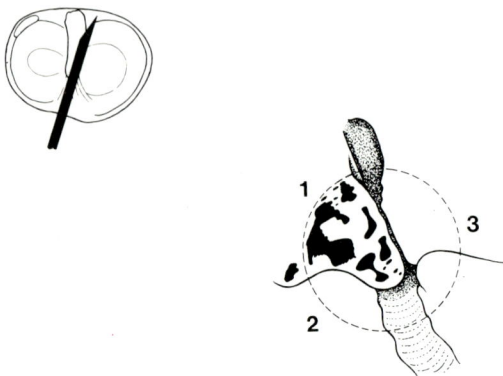

Fig. 2.25 A ruptured posterior cruciate ligament seen with a 70° arthroscope inserted from the antero-lateral approach and passed through the intercondylar notch. The ruptured end of the posterior cruciate ligament (1) is seen lying above the posterior margin of the tibia (2), and anterior to the posterior capsule (3)

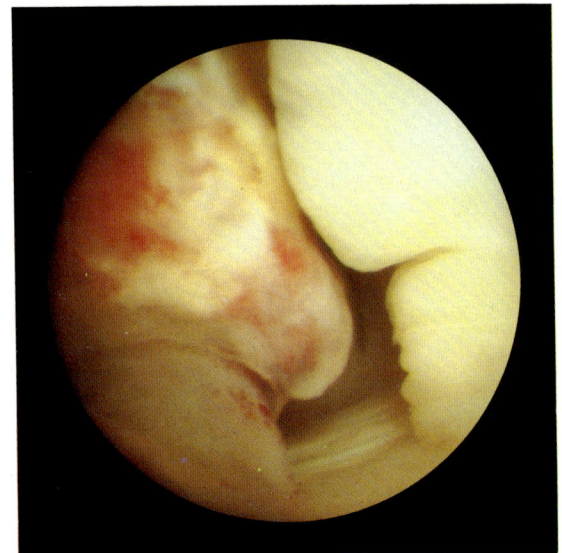

Postero-lateral compartment

The postero-lateral compartment can be entered from the antero-lateral approach in almost every patient by passing the telescope between the lateral femoral condyle and the anterior cruciate ligament in much the same way as the postero-medial compartment is entered. The back of the lateral femoral condyle and the lateral meniscus can then be examined, if necessary by substituting the 70° telescope for the 30°.

Finally, the arthroscope should be brought back to the suprapatellar pouch while plans are laid for the examination of any suspicious areas of special interest with percutaneous needles, the probing hook or a second insertion of the arthroscope.

Other approaches

The central approach

The central approach directly through the patellar tendon (Gillquist and Hagberg 1976) is a practicable alternative to the antero-lateral insertion for the routine initial examination, and offers easier access to the posterior compartments than is usual from the antero-lateral approach. With the knee flexed to 60°, a short skin incision is made in the midline of the knee 1 cm below the lower pole of the patella, down to the patellar tendon but not into it (Fig. 2.9). The trocar is then directed backwards and slightly upwards through the tendon, the fibres of which separate easily

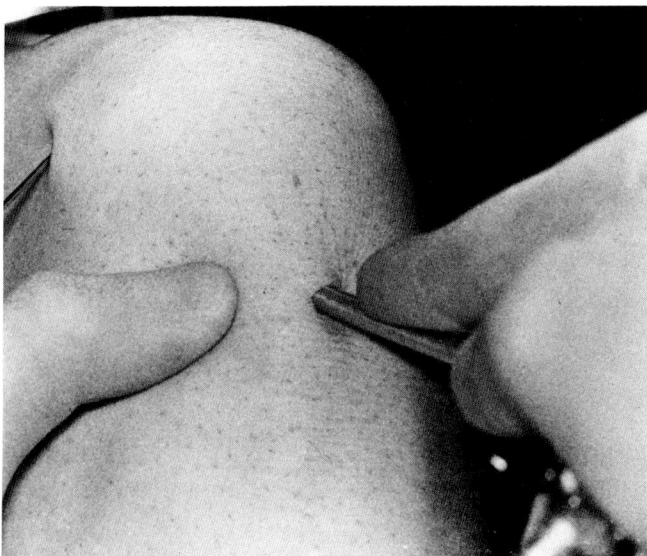

Fig. 2.26 Inserting the trocar of the arthroscope from the central approach

around the shaft of the trocar (Fig. 2.26). The tip of the instrument is then tilted, the knee straightened, and the arthroscope brought into the suprapatellar pouch where the instrument is assembled in the usual way and the joint examined according to the routine already described for the antero-lateral approach. The mobility of the arthroscope is restricted very slightly by the patellar tendon and patella, and examination of the suprapatellar pouch, and in particular the region of the medial shelf, is not as easy from this approach as from the antero-lateral.

The medial compartment can be examined very thoroughly and it is easier to insinuate the tip of the arthroscope between the cruciate ligaments and the medial femoral condyle to enter the postero-medial compartment from this approach than from the antero-lateral. The intercondylar notch and lateral compartment can be examined as thoroughly from this approach as from the antero-lateral, but the lateral gutter, including the popliteus tendon, is less accessible.

The wound and the area of induration in the subcutaneous tissue around it is generally less conspicuous after a central than an antero-lateral or antero-medial approach, perhaps because there is so little subcutaneous tissue overlying the patellar tendon. Although it might seem that to pass a trocar and cannula directly through the patellar tendon is to tempt fate unnecessarily, it must be remembered that the para-patellar approaches involve puncture of the joint capsule, and this may be more traumatic than a simple split along the grain of the patellar tendon.

One minor disadvantage of the central approach is that operating instruments inserted through second and third channels from the antero-medial or antero-lateral routes come to lie very close to the arthroscope. Apart from the undesirability of three wounds so close together, the arthroscope and instruments tend to get in the way of each other and make manipulation difficult. A second disadvantage is that the fibres of the patellar tendon close together so neatly after the arthroscope is withdrawn that it is difficult to find the original passage if the arthroscope is withdrawn either accidentally or intentionally, and repeated insertion of instruments is potentially more harmful through the patellar tendon than through the joint capsule. Despite the simplicity and proven safety of this approach, the author has the fear that if every beginner were to learn arthroscopy from the central approach and use it for routine examination, a patellar tendon will rupture sooner or later and lead to difficulties for both the patient and his surgeon.

Despite these reservations, the central approach has the advantage that it allows two operating instruments to be brought to bear on a meniscal lesion and all surgeons are strongly recommended to become familiar with this approach even if it is not used routinely.

Antero-medial approach

The antero-medial approach has no place as the routine initial insertion for diagnostic arthroscopy. Although the medial side of the patella, medial gutter, postero-medial compartment and anterior horn of the lateral meniscus can be seen better from the medial approach than the lateral, visualisation of the medial synovial shelf, lateral gutter, and anterior part of the medial meniscus is much more difficult and can be virtually impossible if there is a bucket handle fragment of the medial meniscus jammed in the intercondylar notch.

Apart from the limitations of the field of vision, manipulation of an arthroscope inserted on the medial side of the knee is physically clumsy and makes it necessary for the arthroscopist to adopt some curiously contorted postures (Fig. 2.27). Despite these criticisms, a thorough understanding of the antero-medial approach is essential because the antero-medial insertion is the usual route for the operating instruments and cannula when the double puncture technique is

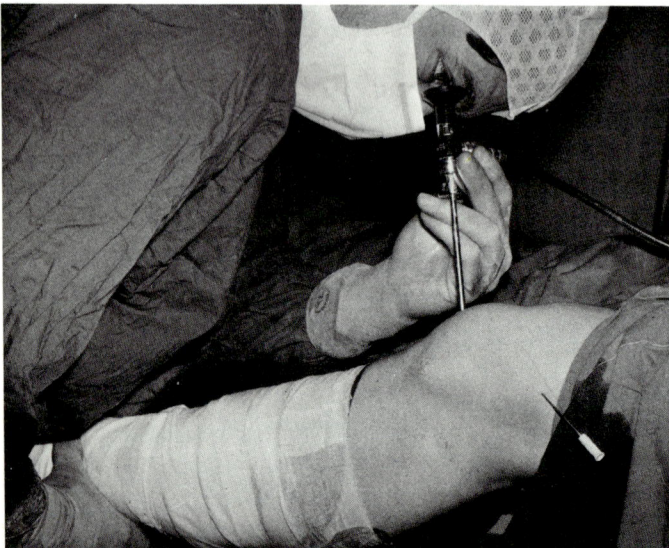

Fig. 2.27 Examining the lateral compartment from the antero-medial approach

used and transposition of the instruments and arthroscope during arthroscopic meniscectomy is often necessary.

The exact point of insertion of the arthroscope is determined by the point at which the operating instruments are to be inserted, which is in turn determined by the anatomy of the lesion to be dealt with and will be described at length in a later chapter. In general, the point of insertion will lie in an area approximately 1 cm above the anterior horn of the medial meniscus and 1.5 cm medial to the patellar tendon (Fig. 2.9). If the point of insertion lies about 1 cm above the medial meniscus, the posterior attachment of the meniscus, the intercondylar notch and lateral meniscus can all be seen easily. The posterior third of the medial meniscus is seen more easily if the insertion is a little lower, while the middle third of the meniscus and the medial gutter are best seen if the arthroscope is inserted 1 cm medial to the edge of the patellar tendon.

Postero-medial insertions

The postero-medial approach affords a view of the postero-medial compartment only, but fulfils the invaluable service of reducing the 'blind area' to a minimum. The posterior aspect of the medial meniscus can be seen well from this approach, as well as the posterior cruciate ligament and the inferior recess. Loose bodies and large flaps of medial meniscus may be discovered that would otherwise have remained hidden. Splits in the body of the meniscus itself are rare and must be distinguished from folds of synovium at the postero-inferior menisco-synovial junction, which can mimic the appearance of a split in the meniscus itself. Although the anterior margin and inferior surface of the posterior horn can be seen from the antero-lateral approach and the posterior surface from the postero-medial approach, it is still possible for small splits in the substance of the meniscus itself to escape detection.

The point of insertion for the postero-medial approach is in the triangle that lies above the tibial plateau and behind the posterior edge of the medial femoral condyle when the knee is flexed to 90°, directly over the pouch of loose capsule and synovium that appears when the knee is flexed (Fig. 2.28). Care should be taken to determine the point of insertion exactly, for if a trocar is placed too far anteriorly it will damage the articular cartilage of the femur and if

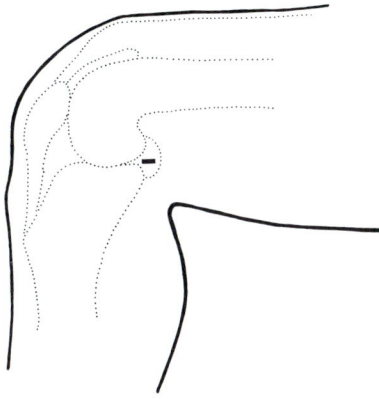

Fig. 2.28 The point of insertion of the arthroscope from the postero-medial approach

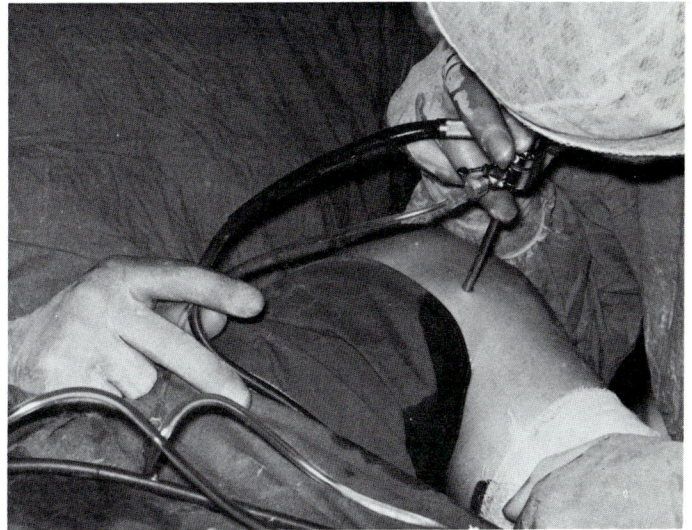

Fig. 2.29 Examining the postero-medial compartment from the postero-medial approach

placed too far posteriorly may lie outside the capsule and endanger the popliteal vessels and nerves. Until familiar with this insertion, it is wise to distend the joint fully with saline with the knee extended, flex the knee to 90°, and insert a needle at the proposed site of insertion. If there is a free flow of saline from the needle the inference may be made that the needle lies in the joint and that the arthroscope can be inserted safely at that point. The trocar can then be inserted through the usual 5 mm horizontal skin incision, aiming slightly upwards and slightly forwards (Fig. 2.29).

The postero-medial compartment is best seen with the knee flexed to 90°, the outer edge of the foot lying on the operating table, and the hip in abduction. The

back of the femoral condyle and meniscus may be examined first unless any loose bodies or meniscal flaps are found lying loose on the floor of the compartment. The synovium covering the cruciate ligaments blocks entry to the lateral compartment, making it impossible for instruments, or loose bodies, to pass directly from the postero-medial to the postero-lateral compartment (Fig. 2.30). A small defect is sometimes seen below the cruciate 'mesentery', but is not large enough to admit the arthroscope and the lateral compartment cannot be entered unless

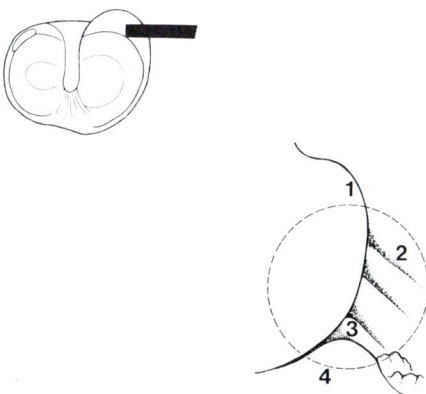

Fig. 2.30 A normal postero-medial compartment from the postero-medial approach; (1) medial femoral condyle (2) posterior capsule (3) posterior cruciate ligament (4) medial meniscus

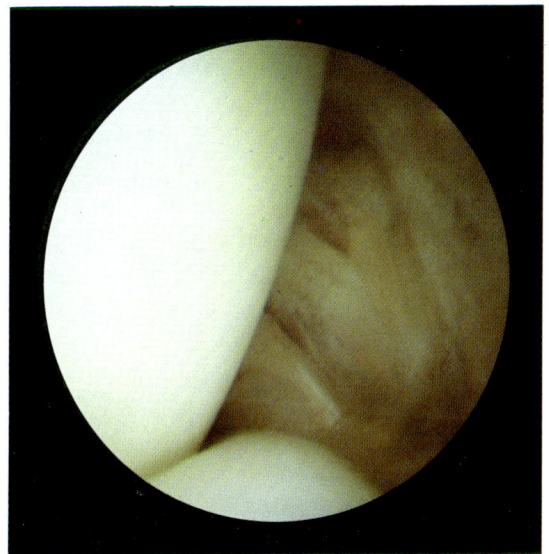

the posterior cruciate ligament is ruptured. Rotating the arthroscope to bring its line of vision posteriorly brings the posterior capsule and its femoral reflection into view but the synovium in this area is usually featureless, apart from the striations of the posterior oblique ligament, with the openings of tunnels leading to popliteal cysts disappointingly absent.

Postero-lateral approach

The postero-lateral compartment can be entered with either the 5 mm or the small diameter arthroscope, but the ilio-tibial tract and capsule in this area are so dense and closely applied to the femur that this insertion is more traumatic than those previously described. This approach reveals nothing that is not seen equally well with the 70° telescope inserted from the antero-lateral or suprapatellar approaches, and is not essential for arthroscopic surgery.

Lateral suprapatellar approach

The lateral suprapatellar approach has greater importance as a route for operating instruments than for the arthroscope itself, but there are occasions when a view from this insertion is helpful in the evaluation of the synovial plicae, lesions of the patella, fat-pad, or the anterior horn of either meniscus (Fig. 2.31). Operative procedures involving the patella, fat-pad, medial shelf or medial meniscus are sometimes completed more easily if the arthroscope is inserted in the suprapatellar pouch with the operating instruments from the antero-medial or antero-lateral route (Fig. 4.13).

Difficulty with this approach may arise if the patient has a deep intercondylar groove and a correspondingly sharp angle between the medial and lateral facets of the patella making it difficult to move the arthroscope easily in the pouch. This difficulty can be avoided by observing the irrigation needle with the arthroscope inserted from the antero-lateral route to be sure that its movement within the pouch is free before removing the needle and replacing it with the arthroscope inserted at the same point. The most convenient point for this insertion is 1 cm posterior to the supero-lateral angle of the patella.

From this route the upper pole of the patella, medial suprapatellar fold, medial synovial shelf and the patello-femoral joint can be seen from above, and the relationship of the shelf and femoral condyle observed. The arthroscope can also be directed downwards into the lateral gutter and the popliteus tendon examined.

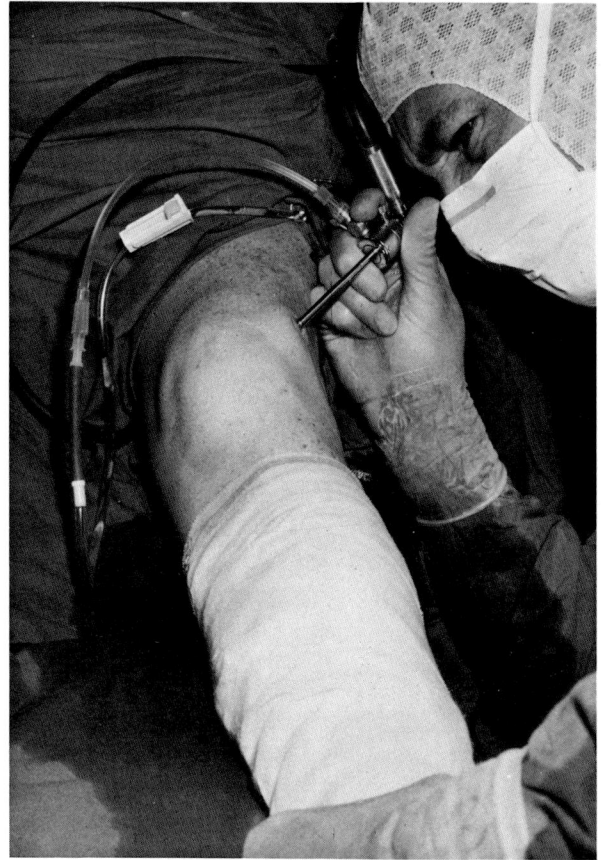

Fig. 2.31 Examining the knee from the suprapatellar approach

An excellent view of the tendon, its tunnel and the postero-lateral compartment is possible with the 70° telescope from this route.

Alternative approaches

The medial suprapatellar approach is sometimes helpful in the release of synovial adhesions or ankylosis, but should only be required exceptionally. The central suprapatellar approach through the quadriceps tendon has no advantage over other approaches and is not needed for arthroscopic surgery.

Probing needles and hooks

The use of the percutaneous needle and blunt hook to manipulate structures within the joint is not only an essential part of the complete arthroscopic examination of the knee, but also constitutes an important phase in the learning of arthroscopy and arthroscopic surgery. The roles of the joint line needle and probing hook in the practical examination of the joint are described below, and their place in the learning of arthroscopic surgery in Chapter 7. It is important to be thoroughly familiar with the use of these instruments before attempting arthroscopic surgery, and those who are unfamiliar with these techniques may find it helpful to study Chapter 7 before proceeding to the basic techniques of arthroscopic surgery outlined in Chapter 3.

Percutaneous needles

The use of percutaneous needles to assess the integrity of the meniscus is simple in principle but slightly more difficult in practice. A No. 21 gauge hypodermic needle is convenient for the purpose and may be placed either beneath the meniscus to sweep out flaps from under the posterior horn and lift the meniscus so that its under-surface can be inspected (Fig. 2.32), or directly into the substance of the meniscus itself to determine whether the rim of the meniscus is stable or detached (Figs. 6.7, 6.8, 6.57, 6.59).

The ideal point of insertion of the needle can be determined by directing the tip of the arthroscope to the desired point of entry and passing the needle through the area of trans-illuminated skin. The first placement of the needle may be a few millimetres off target, but the second attempt should be exact. Random percutaneous stabbing of the meniscus is not to be encouraged. The irrigation needle in the

suprapatellar pouch can also be used to explore the patella, the medial synovial fold or the synovial shelf, and needles at other sites can be used to examine chondral flaps or osteochondritic lesions (Fig. 5.13).

Probing hook

A blunt hook passed through a second channel from the antero-medial approach is invaluable in the assessment of doubtful menisci, lax ligaments (Fig. 2.33), and articular cartilage defects. If the clinical history indicates that a meniscus lesion is possible, the arthroscopic examination is incomplete unless a probing hook is used to test the stability of the posterior third of the meniscus. The hook should be slipped beneath the meniscus and moved with its tip trailing until the doubtful area of meniscus is reached, then turned so that its tip is directed upwards to engage the under-surface of the meniscus and the meniscus pulled forward to test its stability (Fig. 6.9). Like the needle, the hook can also be used to sweep flaps from under the meniscus, to palpate the articular cartilage over areas of osteochondritis dissecans, to assess the integrity of the anterior cruciate ligament, and to determine the full extent of chondral flaps and articular cartilage defects.

Post-operative care and bandaging

A single stitch of mono-filament nylon extending through skin and subcutaneous tissues is the most

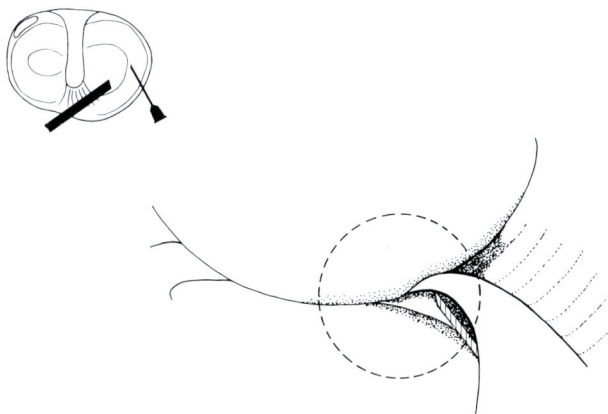

Fig. 2.32 Lifting the medial meniscus with a percutaneous joint line needle to expose its under surface and the inferior coronary ligament

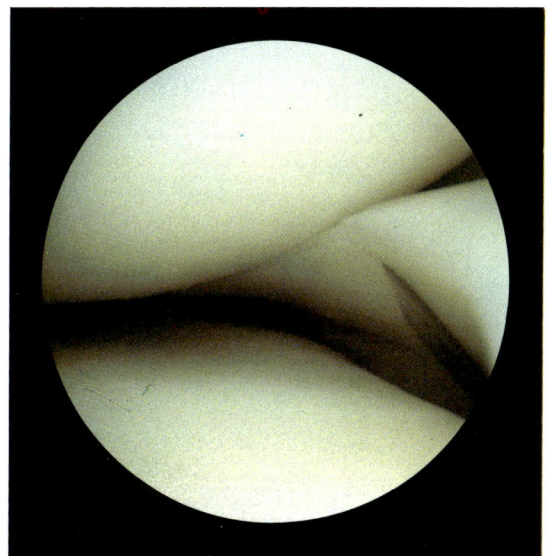

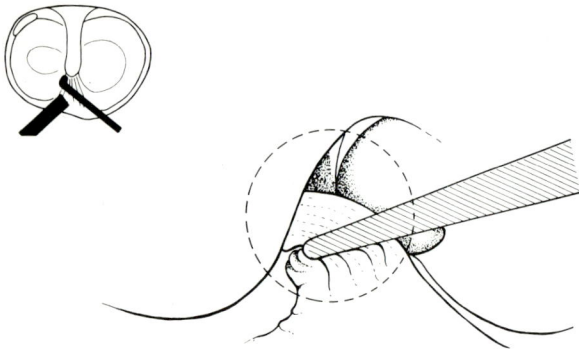

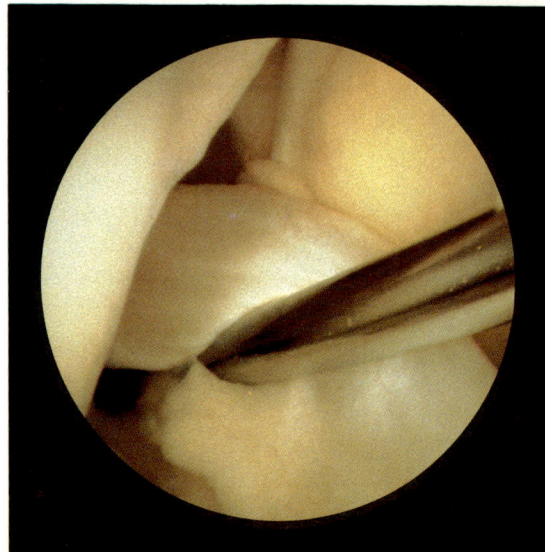

Fig. 2.33 Although this anterior cruciate ligament was apparently intact, the anterior drawer sign was positive and the hook demonstrated abnormal laxity

convenient and effective wound closure. Adhesive tape can also be used for skin closure, but a stitch will close the deeper layers of the wound more effectively and reduce the risk of a haematoma developing at the site of insertion. A subcutaneous stitch and adhesive tape is an alternative, but the subcutaneous stitch will itself lead to an inflammatory reaction which may be more prolonged and uncomfortable than a small haematoma.

When the wound has been closed, a gauze dressing should be applied and the knee supported with a few turns of light orthopaedic wool and a crepe bandage. The bandage should be applied around the knee and not the calf. There is a tendency among nurses and assistants to extend the bandage halfway down the calf—which results in oedema of the ankle and foot—while not taking the bandage to the upper limit of the suprapatellar pouch. The bandage should extend at least 20 cms (8″) above the jointline, and no more than 4 cms (1½″) below it (Fig. 2.34). The patient can expect to raise the leg straight and flex the knee to 90° immediately and to return home either on the same evening or the day after operation, providing that recovery from the effects of the general anaesthetic is complete. The stitch can be removed after seven days. The bandage may be removed on the day after operation if necessary but should be retained for one week if the joint is inflamed.

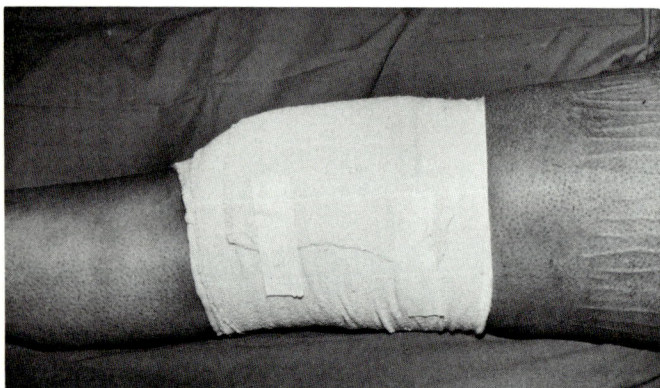

Fig. 2.34 The bandage should extend above the upper limit of the suprapatellar pouch and should not include the calf

REFERENCES

Gillies H, Seligson D 1979 Precision in the Diagnosis of Meniscal Lesions: A Comparison of Clinical Evaluation, Arthrography and Arthroscopy. Journal of Bone and Joint Surgery 61–A: 343–346
Gillquist J, Hagberg G 1976 A New Modification of the Technique of Arthroscopy of the Knee Joint. Acta Chirurgica Scandinavica 142 (2): 123–30
Iino S 1939 Normal Arthroscopic findings in the knee joint in adult Cadavers. Journal of the Japanese Orthopaedic Association 14: 467–523
Jackson R W, Abe I The Role of Arthroscopy in the Management of Disorders of the Knee. Journal of Bone and Joint Surgery 54B: 310–322
Jackson R W, Dandy D J 1976 Arthroscopy of the Knee. Grune & Stratton, New York
Johnson L L 1977 The Comprehensive Examination of the Knee. C V Mosby Co, St. Louis

Johnson L L, Becker R L 1976 Arthroscopy. Technique and the role of the Assistant. Orthopaedic Review 5: 31–43

McGinty J B, Matza R A 1978 Arthroscopy of the Knee. Evaluation of an Out-Patient Procedure under Local Anaesthesia. Journal of Bone and Joint Surgery 60-A: 787–789

Patel D 1978 Arthroscopy of the plicae-synovial folds and their significance. The American Journal of Sports Medicine 6: 217–224

Whipple T L, Bassett F H 1978 Arthroscopic Examination of the Knee. Polypuncture technique with percutaneous intra-articular manipulation. Journal of Bone and Joint Surgery 60-A: 444–452

3

Basic techniques of arthroscopic surgery

Arthroscopic surgery can be performed using the 'double puncture' technique in which operating instruments are inserted through a second cannula separate from the arthroscope, by the 'single puncture' technique using an operating arthroscope that incorporates an extra channel for the operating instruments, or by a combination of both these techniques.

The double and single puncture techniques both have their parts to play in arthroscopic surgery and are not in competition with each other. An operating arthroscope allows instruments to be moved in and out of the knee in a line parallel with the telescope, which is impossible with the double puncture technique, but there are many times when structures must be cut from a different angle and this is only possible through a second channel. The use of an operating arthroscope in conjunction with operating instruments inserted through a separate channel is also possible and is exemplified by the use of grasping forceps inserted through a separate cannula to apply traction to a meniscal fragment which can then be cut from the side with the scissors of the operating arthroscope. Which ever technique is used, three basic rules must be observed:

1. Identify the pathology precisely
2. Plan the approach carefully before inserting the operating instruments
3. Keep the tip of the instruments in view at all times and never cut blindly.

Instruments

Operating arthroscopes

The single puncture technique requires the use of an operating arthroscope, of which there are two basic types. When considering the evolution of the operating arthroscope, it should be remembered that certain instruments started out in life as paediatric cystoscopes, and that some of the 'arthroscopes' still have markings on the barrel at 1 cm intervals to show how far along the urethra the instrument has been passed. These instruments can be fitted with a diathermy lead for electrocoagulation of bladder polyps in place of the bridge on the instrument and these accessories are the reason for the provision of the bridge that now creates so many difficulties, and even dangers, for the arthroscopist who uses such an instrument for diagnostic arthroscopy.

With this type of instrument, the biopsy forceps are inserted by removing the narrower telescope and bridge from the sheath and replacing them with forceps, which then come to lie close to the lens of the telescope at the end of the instrument (Fig. 3.1). This instrument is excellent not only for working inside the bladder but also for synovial biopsy in the suprapatellar pouch, and is probably the arthroscope of choice for the rheumatologist taking specimens of

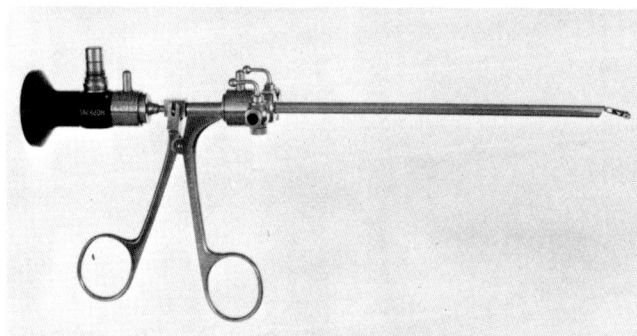

Fig. 3.1 The Storz diagnostic arthroscope with biopsy forceps inserted in place of the bridge

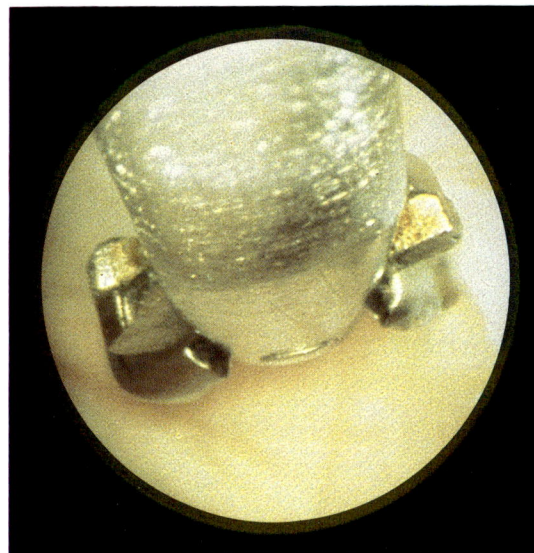

Fig. 3.2 The view down the Storz diagnostic arthroscope with the biopsy forceps in position

synovium for histological study. Sadly, such a simple instrument is of little use in other procedures for several reasons, of which the greatest is the fixed position of the biopsy forceps at the end of the telescope. Because of their position, the forceps will only cut structures that can be brought flat against the end of the instrument, and cannot be brought to bear upon structures such as the posterior horn of the medial meniscus and cannot be removed from the knee without removing the telescope as well. Secondly, while quite adequate for removing 1–2 mm diameter fragments of vesical polyps or inflamed synovium the forceps are simply not strong enough to make any impression on the average meniscus. Difficulties also arise from the use of the narrow telescope which has a narrower angle of vision than the thicker telescope used in the diagnostic instruments and affords a smaller field of view, much of which is obscured by the forceps (Fig. 3.2).

Because of these difficulties, operating arthroscopes have been developed with a separate instrument channel through which the instruments can be moved in and out of the knee parallel with the telescope so that tight areas can be entered with ease and structures cut at some distance from the lens. The introduction of an instrument channel parallel with the telescope makes it necessary to move the eyepiece well away from the instrument channel and in the most widely used operating arthroscope, developed by Dr R L O'Connor in association with the Wolf Company, this

is achieved by adding two 90° bends to the lens system (Fig. 3.3). The O'Connor/Wolf operating arthroscope uses a narrow telescope with a smaller field of vision than that used in the diagnostic instrument, and includes two irrigation channels as well as a glass fibre light guide. The resulting instrument has an outside diameter of 6.5 mm and is more bulky than most diagnostic arthroscopes but the Stryker Company have recently introduced a new operation arthroscope developed by Dr R W Carson, in which the two 90° bends are omitted and the bulk of the instrument is reduced further by enclosing the operating instruments and telescope in a tube of oval section.

A little practice is required before an operating arthroscope can be handled with ease (Fig. 3.4). The main problems encountered in its use are difficulty in manipulating the instrument because of its bulk, the fragility of the 3 mm cutting instruments, and the reduced field of vision from the narrow telescope

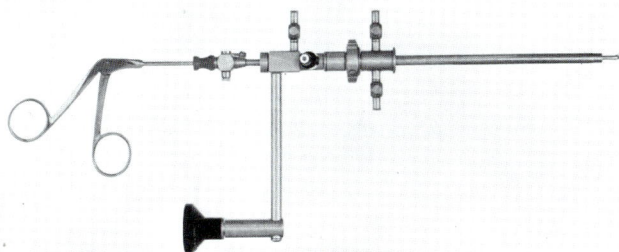

Fig. 3.3 The Wolf operating arthroscope with the scissors in the instrument channel

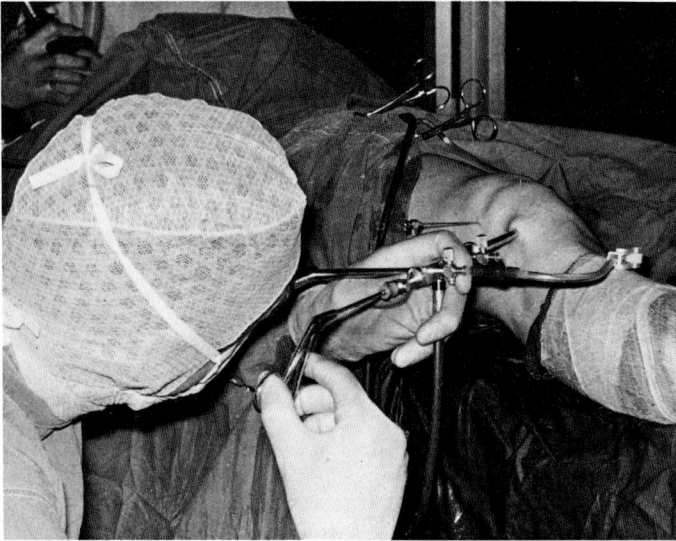

Fig. 3.4 Using the Wolf operating arthroscope to excise the medial synovial shelf

which make orientation difficult when the telescope is close to its target. This problem can be eased by identifying the target area from a distance, touching it with a tip of an operating instrument advanced through the instrument channel, and 'railroading' the arthroscope along the operating instrument.

The operating instruments supplied with the operating arthroscopes include grasping forceps, basket forceps, and a selection of knives (Fig. 3.5).

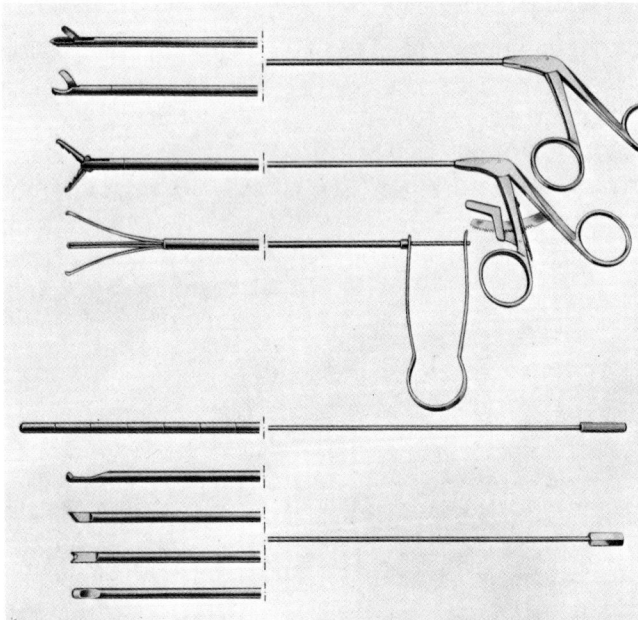

Fig. 3.5 Instruments for the Wolf operating arthroscope. From above downwards; basket forceps, scissors, grasping forceps, spring-loaded grasping forceps, probe, and four knives

Meniscal tissue can be divided satisfactorily with the scissors as long as the tissue is snipped in little bites but both scissors and basket forceps quickly lose their cutting edge if used on meniscal tissue and need either to be resharpened or replaced after some thirty or forty procedures.

The operating arthroscope is a very useful instrument for a variety of operations notably the division of the synovial shelf and other soft tissue procedures in the suprapatellar pouch, but stronger cutting or grasping instruments inserted through a second channel are required for other procedures. An operating arthroscope is by no means essential for the practice of arthroscopic surgery, but its use simplifies many procedures.

Double puncture technique

It is quite possible to operate inside the knee using standard instruments found in any well-equipped operating theatre, and to remove a locked bucket handle fragment of medial meniscus using only a tenotomy knife and a pair of pituitary rongeurs, but the use of specially designed instruments extends the range of operations and makes them simpler. Although instruments are already available in most operating theatres for laparoscopy and other endoscopic procedures, the special requirements of cutting tough meniscal tissue inside the narrow potential space of the knee rather than soft tissue in a cavern such as the bladder or abdomen make laparoscopic instruments unsuitable for work within the knee.

The most important requirement for operating instruments in this kind of surgery is that they must be both strong enough to cut meniscal tissue without bending or breaking and small enough to be manipulated easily inside the knee. Instruments such as scissors or grasping forceps with jaws that open inside the joint must be small enough to be opened in the intercondylar notch and strong enough to cut meniscal tissue, requirements which are almost impossible to reconcile. There is no need for the instruments to be circular in section, and oval instruments have the advantage of being more easily manoeuvrable without a corresponding loss of strength.

Bow handles should be avoided because firm pressure of the surgeon's thumb against the side of the bow can damage the cutaneous nerve of the thumb at the level of the proximal phalanx (Fig. 3.6). In the author's experience, such lesions take between two

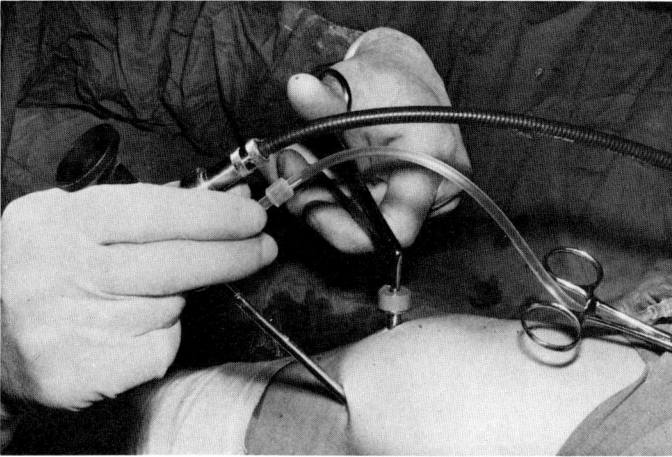

Fig. 3.6 Double puncture technique. The forceps are held wrongly with the surgeon's thumb passed completely through the bow of the handle

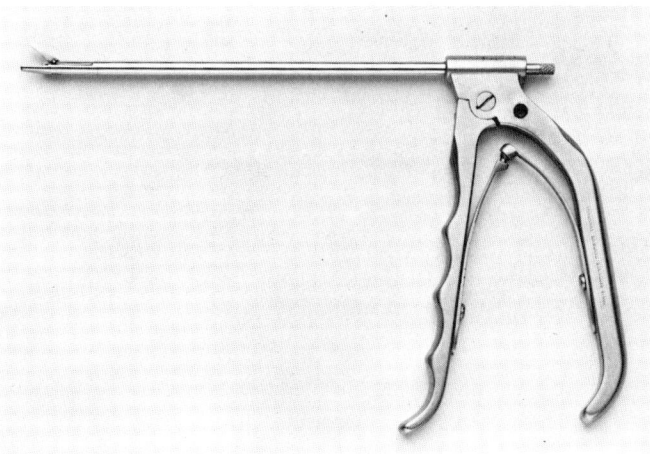

Fig. 3.8 Tips of the Thackray operating instruments. From above downwards; punch forceps, scissors, and guillotine

and twelve weeks to resolve. Although altered sensibility of the skin along the edge of the thumb is only a minor inconvenience, it is nevertheless worth avoiding by the use of handles that are specifically designed for gripping and do not include a metal ring for the thumb (Fig. 3.7).

The instruments must also be designed so that their tips are free of sharp edges or corners and will run smoothly over the articular cartilage without causing damage (Fig. 3.8), and it is helpful if the profile of the tip is so shaped that it can be passed easily along the track of the instrument cannula if the cannula is withdrawn either accidentally or intentionally. Finally, it is helpful if the instruments, which are all superficially similar, can be identified quickly and easily by the scrub nurse or assistant in a darkened operating theatre by some device such as coloured markers or notches on the handle of the instrument.

The basic set of operating instruments includes a trocar and cannula, a probing hook, a knife (Fig. 3.9), straight and curved pituitary rongeurs, grasping forceps, punch forceps, scissors and a guillotine (Fig. 3.10). Although this set of instruments will usually be sufficient, there are occasions when a variety of other instruments may be required, including a sharp skin hook, a pair of tendon tunnelling forceps, and an assortment of tools originally intended for surgery of the ear, nose and throat or other endoscopic procedures (Fig. 3.11).

The outside diameter of the instruments should be no greater than that of the standard diagnostic arthroscope (5 mm). Round barrelled instruments are passed into the joint through a cannula with an outside diameter of 6 mm, itself introduced over a trocar 5 mm in diameter, and the curved flat instruments along the track of the cannula after it has been removed. The 6 mm cannula has the advantage that

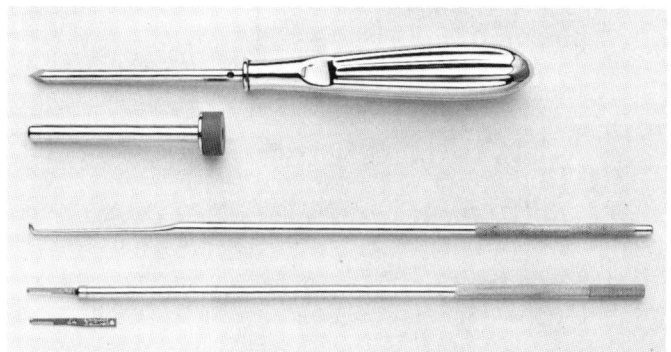

Fig. 3.7 An overall view of the Thackray operating scissors

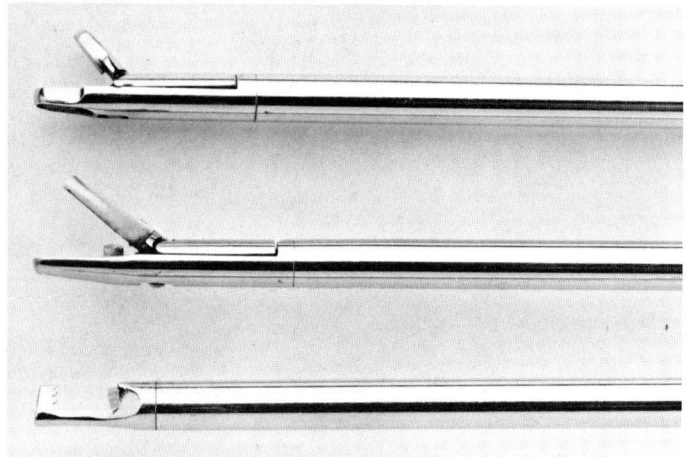

Fig. 3.9 Instruments for double puncture. From above downwards; trocar, cannula with rubber seal, probing hook, long-handled knife, and disposable No. 64 Beaver blade

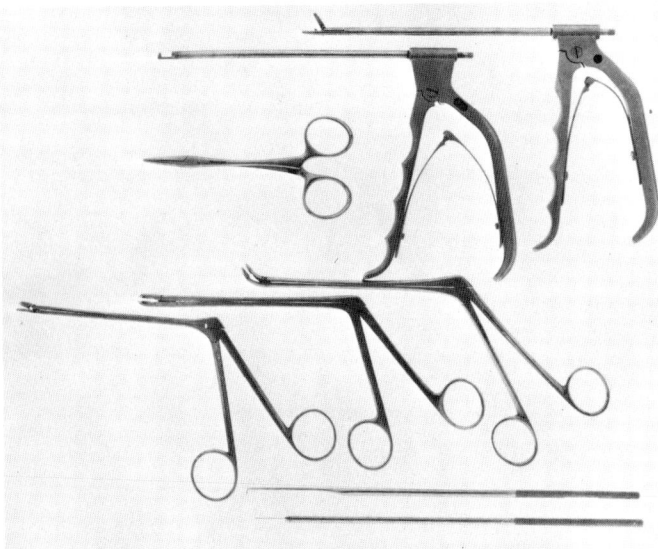

Fig. 3.10 Basic set of instruments for double puncture technique. From above downwards: arthroscopic scissors, guillotine, artery forceps with screw joint, Northfield's curved pituitary rongeurs, Cushing's straight pituitary rongeurs with 4 mm bite, punch forceps, hook and knife

it will admit the arthroscope as well, simplifying the transposition of arthroscope and instruments.

Scissors and basket forceps with a curved shaft that will follow the margin of the meniscus are available with a diameter of 3 mm but, like the instruments of the operating arthroscope, they have the disadvantage that the blades need to be resharpened after thirty or forty procedures. A knife with a retractable blade is also available, but this also requires regular sharpening, a disadvantage that can be overcome by using a simple long handled knife with a disposable blade.

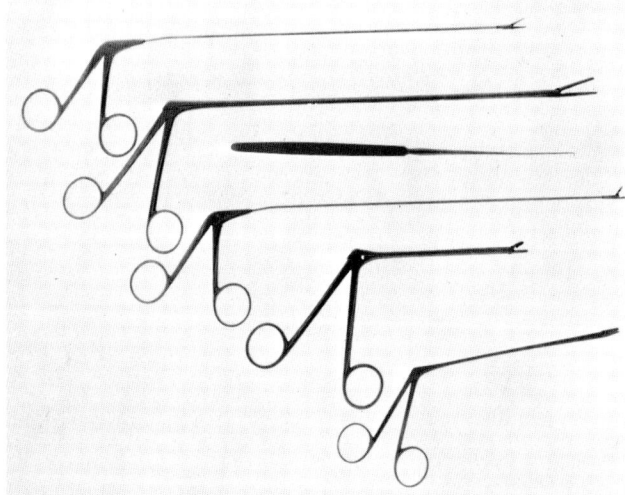

Fig. 3.11 Useful additions to the basic set of instruments. Micro-laryngeal forceps, sigmoidoscopic grasping forceps, modified Gillies' skin-hook, micro-laryngeal cup forceps, punch scissors, and flat nasal scissors

Powered instruments

Apart from simple cutting instruments, powered instruments have also been developed. The original powered instrument for intra-articular surgery was the patellar shaver conceived by Dr Lanny Johnson and made by the Dyonics Corporation (Fig. 3.12). The instrument consists of a hollow tube containing a cylindrical blade that revolves slowly within the tube and cuts tissue drawn into it by gentle suction applied to the handle of the instrument. The cylindrical blade is driven by a small battery-powered motor controlled by a foot-pedal. The shaver is most effective in removing flakes of articular cartilage and other irregularities on the surface of the patella and femoral condyles and can produce not only a very pleasing arthroscopic appearance (Fig. 5.18), but also can be used for synovectomy and 'contouring' the irregular surfaces of damaged menisci. The shaver is also an effective, albeit expensive, vacuum-cleaner for removing debris from the knee.

Recent additions to the range of powered instruments include shaving heads only 3 mm wide and a variety of end cutting instruments intended for the removal of meniscal fragments, as well as an instrument with a reciprocating instead of a revolving blade designed for synovectomy. These adaptations are certainly more effective for removing meniscal fragments than the original side cutting shaver, but they must be used with extreme caution.

Although powered instruments may well prove to have a place in arthroscopic surgery, they are by no means an essential or basic piece of equipment and the surgeon is strongly recommended not to purchase the shaver until he has come to the limit of that which can be achieved using simple hand instruments. At the time of writing, powered instruments are surgical novelties and are being used excessively.

Preparation

Arthroscopic operations generally follow a preliminary diagnostic arthroscopy and the comments made in the previous chapter on the use of a tourniquet and the advantages of a general anaesthetic still apply. Arthroscopic surgery without a tourniquet is quite permissible if that is the surgeon's preference, but the beginner will find that the operation is easier if the leg is elevated and a tourniquet inflated. Similarly, local anaesthetic is completely acceptable for certain pro-

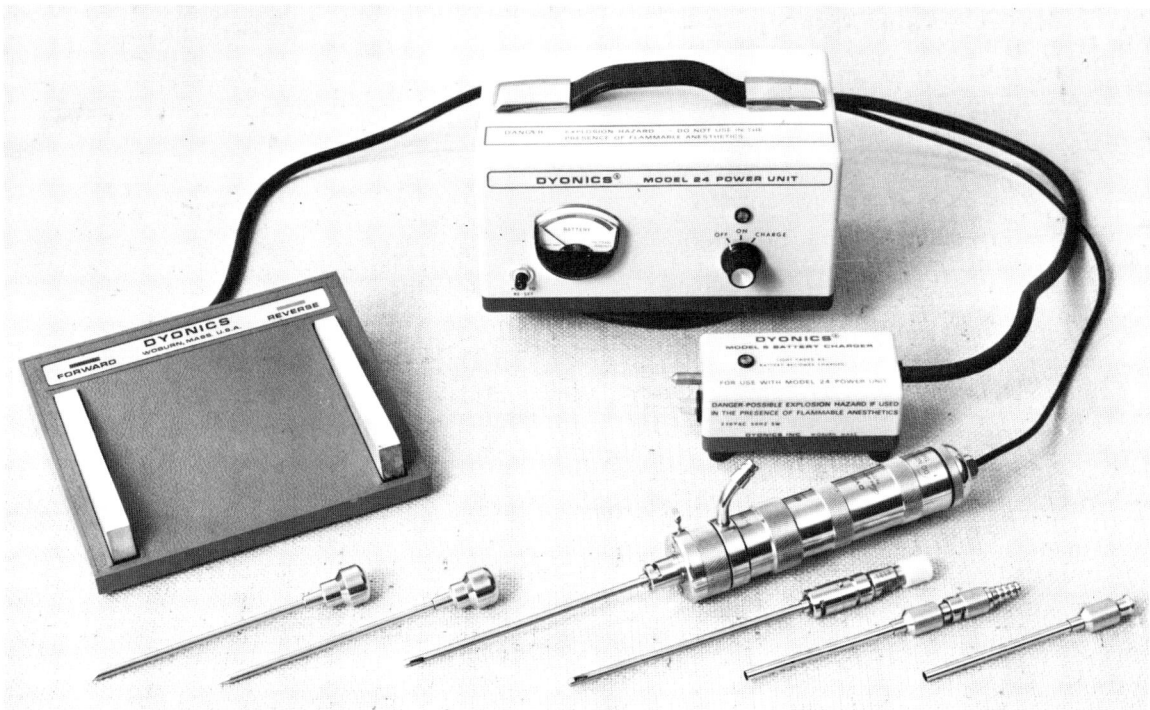

Fig. 3.12 Dyonics shaver with foot pedal, power unit, battery charger, sharp trocar, blunt obturator, shaving attachment and cannula

cedures, particularly those that only involve synovium, but it is sensible for the surgeon to operate under general anaesthesia until he has perfected his technique. If local anaesthetic is to be used, the skin at the points of insertion of the instruments should be infiltrated with 0.5 per cent bupivacaine without added adrenaline and 10 mls of 0.5 lignocaine and 10 mls of 0.5 per cent bupivacaine hydrochloride run into the synovial cavity. The local anaesthetic may be retained in the knee by operating without an irrigation outflow needle, and a tourniquet should not be used (McGinty and Matza 1978).

Whether general or local anaesthesia is used, the patient should be well instructed in quadriceps exercises before operation, and omission of this simple step can delay recovery.

Theatre layout

The layout of the theatre for the initial arthroscopy has already been described and needs little alteration when the operating instruments are used. If both the nurse and the surgeon have considerable experience of arthroscopic surgery, the instrument trolley should stay on the side of the table opposite the surgeon, who can then ask for the instruments by name (Fig. 2.7). In the early days the operation will proceed more

smoothly if the instrument trolley is brought round the table to stand beside the surgeon so that he can help himself to the instruments. The surgeon will also require a stool on which to sit, preferably one with wheels or metal feet for easier manoeuvrability rather than non-slip rubber feet.

Irrigation

The steady flow of irrigation fluid from the tip of the arthroscope to the exit needle in the suprapatellar pouch may be insufficient to remove the debris from some procedures, making it necessary to flush the joint thoroughly clear of debris from time to time. Irrigation is seldom a problem with the double puncture technique because the flow of saline along the instrument cannula is more than adequate, but without a second channel the telescope will need to be removed from its sheath and the joint irrigated by judicious use of the inflow stopcock and a thumb over the end of the sheath. The outflow of saline may be excessive rather than deficient and it is by no means unusual for the surgeon's trousers to be thoroughly soaked by the end of the procedure. This minor embarrassment can be avoided if a waterproof apron is worn under the gown for all procedures but spillage is minimal in many arthroscopies and routine use of an apron is unnecessary as well as uncomfortable and uneconomic.

Double puncture technique

Insertion of the instruments

The trocar and cannula are inserted through a short incision, just as the arthroscopic trocar and cannula are inserted, at a point dictated by the lesion to be treated. The points of insertion are essentially the same as those for the arthroscope described in the previous chapter, and the exact points of insertion for the management of individual lesions will be described later. Attempts to insert the instruments at other sites are inadvisable and likely to damage the articular cartilage of the femur. In particular, the instruments should never be inserted more than 2 cms from the edge of the patellar tendon when using the antero-medial or antero-lateral approach because there is simply not enough space beyond these points either to insert the instrument easily or to manipulate it in the knee without damage to the articular cartilage.

Care must be taken to avoid striking the tip of the arthroscope when the trocar is inserted (Fig. 3.13)—a risk that is greatest when the arthroscope has already been inserted from the antero-lateral route and the instruments are then inserted from the antero-medial route. This mishap can be avoided by inserting the trocar with the knee flexed, and with the arthroscope lying so that its tip points downwards and backwards in the intercondylar notch. The patient's foot can then be rested on the surgeon's knee and the arthroscope

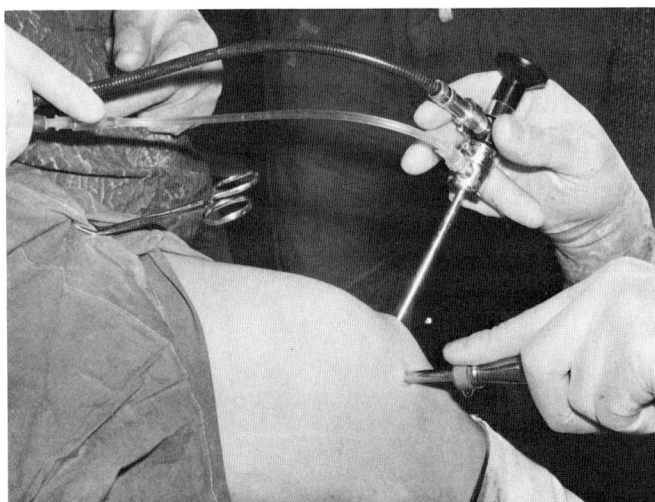

Fig. 3.13 Inserting the cannula for the operating instruments from the antero-medial approach

steadied by an assistant while the trocar is inserted through the usual short skin incision and aimed upwards, backwards and laterally towards the lateral femoral condyle so that it passes well above the arthroscope. When the instruments are to be inserted from the lateral suprapatellar approach the knee should be straight, and the trocar aimed well away from the end of the arthroscope.

When the cannula is in place, the trocar is withdrawn. A gush of saline indicates that the joint has been entered; if the saline does not flow, either the cannula is not in the joint at all or it is so far in that the tip is jammed against the far side of the synovial cavity. The cannula should then be manipulated, if necessary after reinsertion of the trocar, until there is a good flow of saline which is then controlled with a finger, spigot, or an operating instrument.

Manipulating the leg

The importance of holding and manipulating the leg correctly during diagnostic arthroscopy has already been mentioned and is equally important during arthroscopic surgery, in order that the joint space can be opened to give easy access to the different compartments of the knee. With one hand occupied steadying the arthroscope and the other holding operating instruments, manipulation of the leg is even more difficult than it is for diagnostic arthroscopy. One solution is to liberate one hand by holding the arthroscope steady with a modified brain retractor bandaged to the patient's leg, a device which is only partly successful because the position of the arthroscope needs frequent fine adjustment. An alternative is to ask an assistant either to steady the arthroscope or to operate the instruments but without being able to look down the arthroscope himself, the task of the assistant is difficult if not impossible. A modified shoulder rest can also be fixed to the operating table to act as a fulcrum against which the knee can be stressed, but the simplest and most practical answer to the problem is for the surgeon to steady the patient's foot between his own knees and to apply whatever stresses he wishes by appropriate pressure with his hand or knee or by varying the height of the operating table. Although the various manoeuvres seem clumsy at first, with perseverance they will come naturally and without conscious thought.

Sitting on a wheeled stool and with the patient's foot resting on the lap, the knee can be flexed or

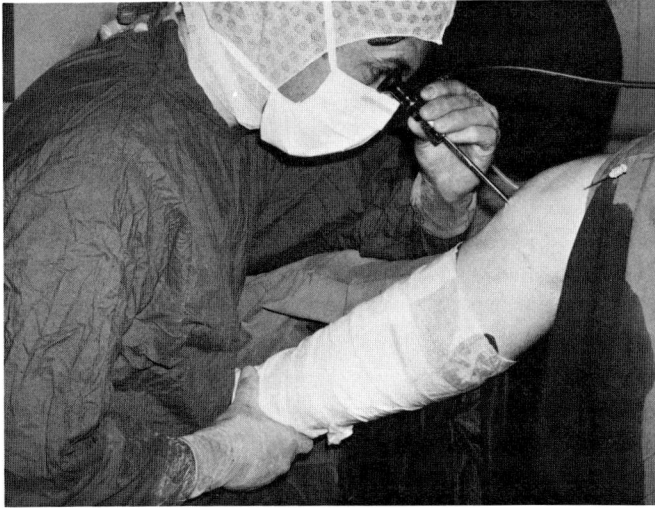

Fig. 3.14 Examining the knee in slight flexion with a varus stress

extended either by movement of the stool towards or away from the patient (Fig. 3.14), or by raising or lowering the operating table. When the right knee is being examined, a valgus stress can be applied if the surgeon sits with his right leg crossed over his left to steady the patient's foot against the inner edge of his right thigh, and then applies the inner aspect of his left forearm to the outer side of the patient's calf (Fig. 3.15). The knee can be rotated internally or externally by movement of the patient's foot (Fig. 3.16). A gentle varus stress is applied by pressure with the hand and wrist against the medial side of the knee and a firmer pressure by using the edge of the operating table as a fulcrum and leaning gently against the outer side of the patient's ankle (Fig. 3.17). Although it is easy to

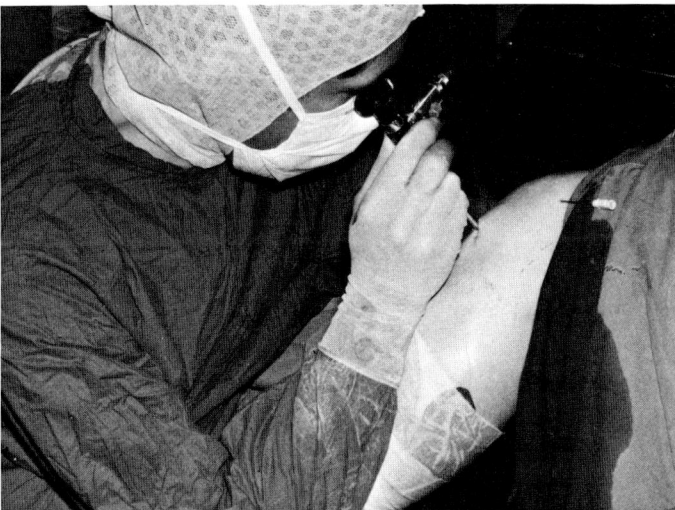

Fig. 3.16 External rotation of the leg

describe how these manipulations are performed, only practice will bring confidence and skill.

Manipulating the instruments and 'triangulation'

The coordinated manipulation of an operating instrument and an arthroscope inserted from two separate points has become known as 'triangulation', and

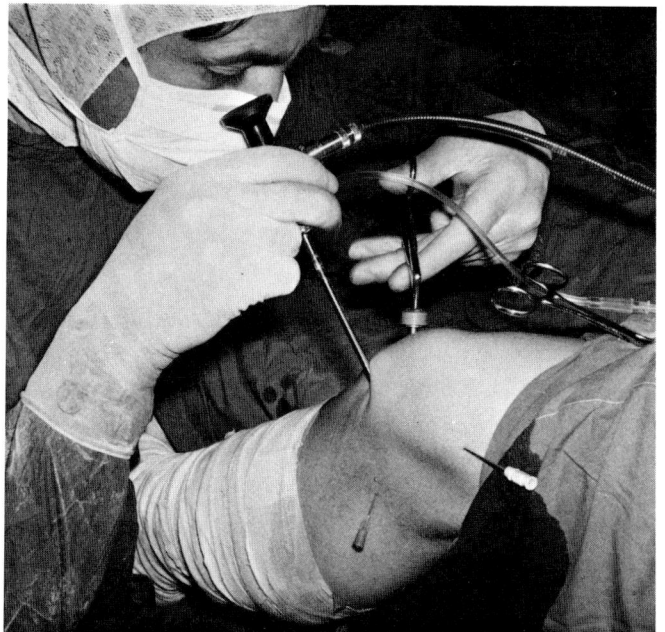

Fig. 3.15 Applying a valgus and external stress without an assistant

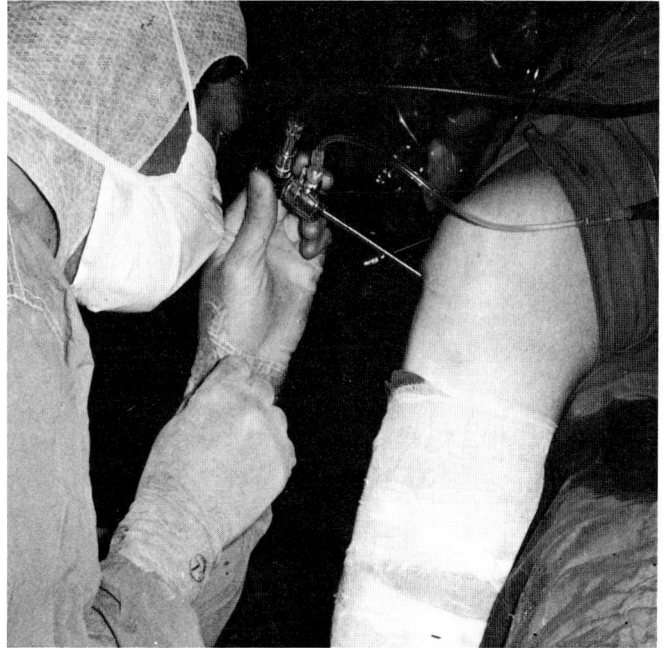

Fig. 3.17 Applying a varus strain while operating in the lateral compartment. The punch forceps are held correctly

forms the basis of the double puncture technique. To direct the tip of an operating instrument held in one hand under the control of an arthroscope held in the other while manipulating the patient's leg with movements of the knees and body is a skill that is not acquired instantly. At first, it is difficult enough to find the tip of the irrigating needle in the suprapatellar pouch without trying to keep it in sight while it is moved from one side of the suprapatellar pouch to the other. It is of no consolation at this stage to know that movement of the instruments in the suprapatellar pouch is considerably easier than in the intercondylar notch or in the medial of lateral compartment, but the beginner may rest assured that just as arthroscopy became straightforward with practice, so will the technique of arthroscopic surgery.

Until the cerebellum has acquired the necessary pathways to find the tip of the operating instruments without conscious effort, one of several other methods of location may be used. The simplest is to look away from the eyepiece and place the tip of the instrument in front of the telescope by pointing the shafts of the instruments towards each other (Figs. 3.6, 3.18). An alternative is to feel the barrel of one instrument with the other and then to slide the barrel of one along to the tip of the other and a third method is to use some easily identifiable point in the knee, such as the intercondylar notch or the apex of the suprapatellar pouch, as a 'reporting base' where the instruments can be placed for easy identification. As with routine diagnostic arthroscopy, orientation of the instrument within the knee is easier with the straight ahead 0° telescope than with the 30°, and the 0° telescope is recommended for use in the early stages of learning the technique of triangulation.

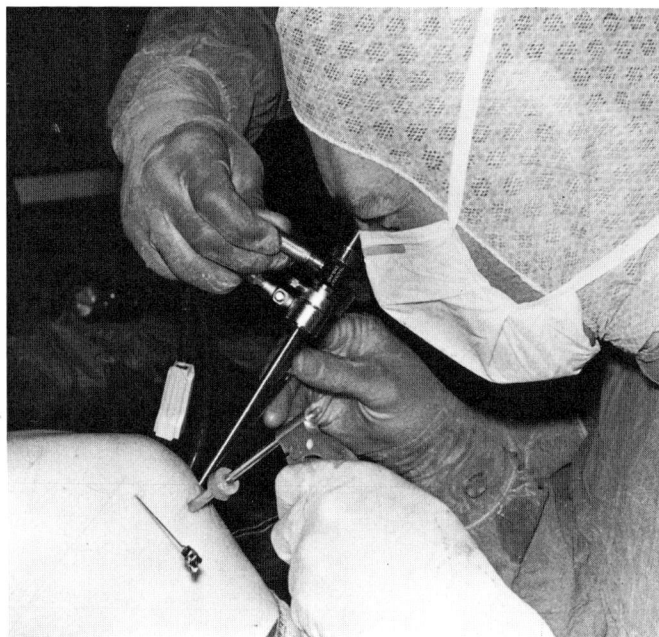

Fig. 3.19 Triple puncture technique with the arthroscope inserted from the central approach. Note the third hand

Triangulation with the arthroscope and one set of instruments is difficult, but the manipulation of an arthroscope from the central approach and one instrument through each of the antero-lateral and antero-medial approaches demands either a third arm or a skilled assistant (Fig. 3.19). Although the use of three approaches simultaneously complicates the procedure, the manipulation of two instruments as well as the arthroscope is sometimes unavoidable and is a skill that must be learned.

A number of basic rules should be observed when handling instruments inside the knee. Firstly, never use cutting instruments unless the tip of the instrument is in full view of the arthroscope and the structure to be cut has been identified beyond any shadow of doubt. Secondly, do not try to take large bites of tissue, particularly meniscus, or the instrument will break (Fig. 8.1). There is a characteristic and easily recognisable 'springy' feel to an instrument that is overloaded; when the instrument does not cut cleanly or feels overloaded, it should be pulled back slightly and a smaller bite of tissue taken. Thirdly, do not twist the operating instruments unnecessarily because twisting stresses are particularly harmful to the hinge mechanism. Finally, as in other fields of surgery, it is important to be as gentle as possible with all tissues, not only to articular cartilage and cruciate ligaments, but to the synovium as well.

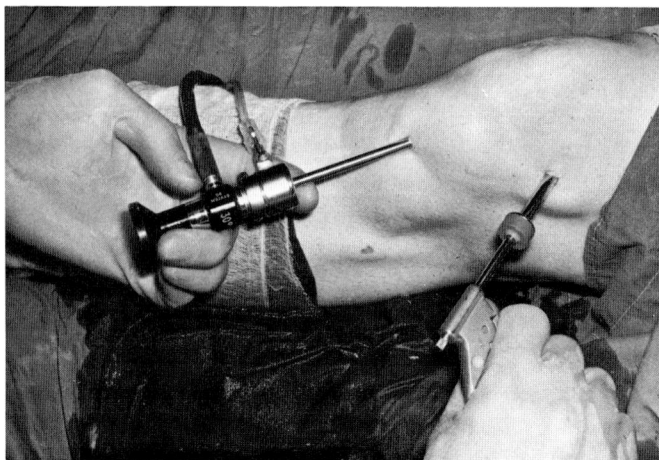

Fig. 3.18 Triangulation in the suprapatellar pouch

Technical problems

Extravasation of fluid

When the double puncture technique is used, irrigation fluid tends to escape from the joint into the subsynovial tissues along the line of the instrument cannula. The amount of fluid that escapes varies according to the pressure of saline within the knee and may be minimised by lowering the irrigation reservoir to reduce the hydrostatic pressure. This manoeuvre, while effective in reducing the outflow of saline, has the disadvantage that the consequent deflation of the joint makes the operation slightly more difficult.

Escape of fluid is particularly troublesome after the suprapatellar insertion of instruments, and also occurs if the synovium is breached by taking a large biopsy specimen, a wide excision of a synovial shelf, or performing a lateral release. For this reason, procedures in the suprapatellar pouch should be planned carefully and concluded as quickly as possible. Although a large collection of subcutaneous saline is harmless and will disappear within 12 hours of operation, it is a minor insult to the tissues and worth avoiding for this reason alone, quite apart from the unpleasing appearance of a swollen and shapeless knee at the end of the procedure (Fig. 3.20).

Synovial fat-pad

The infrapatellar fat-pad is a formidable enemy if distended with saline or engorged with oedema. Extra synovial injection of saline resulting from incorrect placement of the irrigation needle has already been mentioned, and the same problem arises if the tip of the arthroscope is accidentally withdrawn from the synovial cavity and comes to lie in the subcutaneous tissues. The flow of saline from the end of the arthroscope will then run into the surrounding tissues, and the intercondylar notch will quickly become stuffed with a soggy mass of wet tissue which obscures vision completely.

An intense inflammatory response can cause a similar problem (Fig. 3.21). If a patient exercises vigorously with a knee that has been locked with a displaced bucket handle fragment of meniscus for several weeks, the surgeon can confidently expect to find a mass of inflamed synovium obstructing his view of the meniscus and is wise to advise such a patient to take life easily and perhaps to take an anti-inflamma-

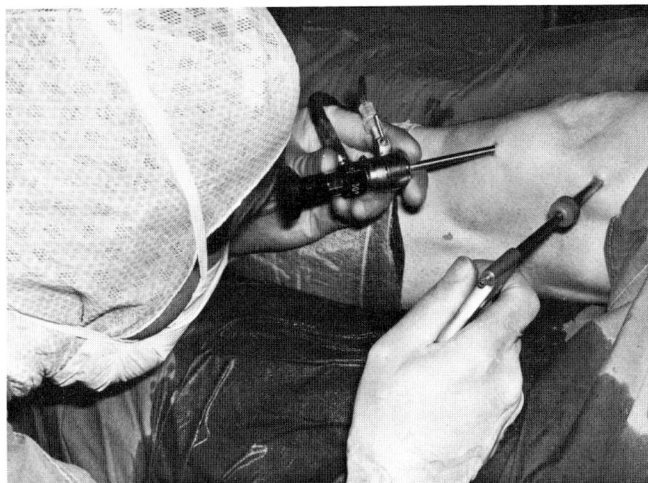

Fig. 3.20 Operating in the suprapatellar pouch. Saline has escaped into the subsynovial tissues to cause an unsightly distension of the subcutaneous tissue

tory drug for a few days before operation so that the engorged tissues will have time to subside.

Apart from incorrect placement of the irrigation needle and an intense inflammatory reaction, operative trauma may cause oedema of the fat-pad, and is made worse by saline tracking outwards along the barrel of the instrument. Swelling of the tissues in the intercondylar notch is sometimes apparent after only 20 or 30 minutes of intra-articular surgery and it is therefore sensible to waste as little time as possible on photography or teaching before dealing with structures in this vulnerable area, and to avoid poking instruments about in the fat-pad any more than is absolutely necessary.

Attempts to design retractors for the fat-pad have so far been unrewarding, and the simple manoeuvre of passing a tape from the antero-medial to antero-lateral approach has also proved unhelpful. The best answer to the problem of the enlarging fat-pad, which is also the most difficult answer, is swift but gentle surgery that is over before the swelling has had time to develop.

Post-operative care

When the intra-articular procedure is completed, the tourniquet should be released and the joint irrigated thoroughly until the effluent is clear. The wounds are then each closed with one nylon stitch (Fig. 3.22), and a dressing of gauze, orthopaedic wool and a crepe bandage applied. Whatever the procedure, patients can expect to lift the leg straight on recovering from

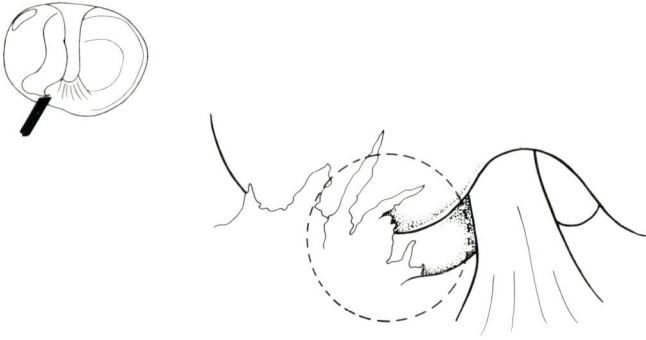

Fig. 3.21 Intense synovitis obscuring a locked bucket handle fragment of the lateral meniscus

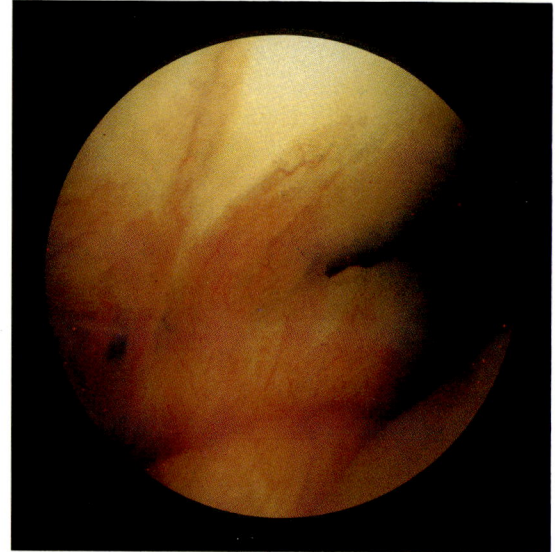

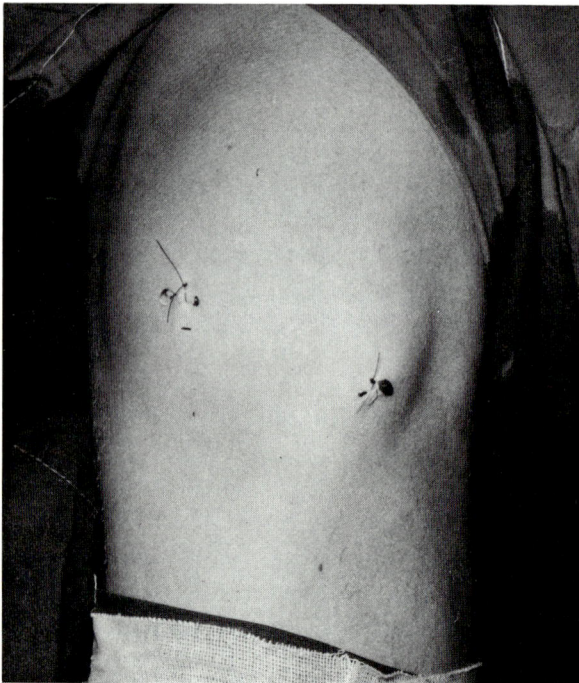

Fig. 3. 22 Wound closure with two nylon stitches after medial meniscectomy

the anaesthetic and to leave hospital either on the day of operation or the day after, provided they have received pre-operative instruction in quadriceps exercises. The post-operative course is a little slower than that which follows arthroscopy alone and, when both antero-medial and antero-lateral approaches have been used, may be associated with swelling and discomfort around the wounds that can make full extension of the knee uncomfortable for a few days.

Post-operative physiotherapy is helpful but not mandatory. Ultra-sound treatment to the wounds may help to speed the natural resolution of the swelling around them, and instruction in quadriceps strengthening exercises is never out of place. Although flexion to 90° is almost always possible within 24 hours of operation, flexion exercises should be avoided for the first week to minimise the risk of persistent synovial effusion. The risk of a low grade chronic synovitis and persistent effusion following early mobilisation of a knee that has been injured either surgically or otherwise is real, and this risk may be reduced by the administration of a non-steroidal anti-inflammatory drug. It is the author's practice to prescribe ketoprofen 50 mgs three times a day or an appropriate dose of a comparable drug for one week after operation and for one or two days before if there is evidence of chronic synovitis.

REFERENCE

McGinty J B, Matza R A 1978 Arthroscopy of the Knee. Evaluation of an Out-Patient Procedure under Local Anesthesia. Journal of Bone and Joint Surgery 60A: 787–789.

4

Operations on synovium and joint capsule

Because synovial biopsy is the simplest arthroscopic procedure and the first to become a routine procedure, the surgeon will probably become familiar with operations involving the synovium before attempting to remove loose bodies or damaged menisci.

Pathological synovium can be assessed more accurately if the knee is examined without a tourniquet, which alters the vascularity of the tissues. The inflation of a tourniquet should therefore be omitted if the appearance of the synovium is likely to be important but, because inflamed synovium is friable and bleeding from it may obscure vision, it is wise to apply a pneumatic tourniquet to the thigh before draping the limb so that if haemorrhage becomes troublesome the leg can be elevated, the tourniquet inflated and the joint irrigated until a clear view is obtained.

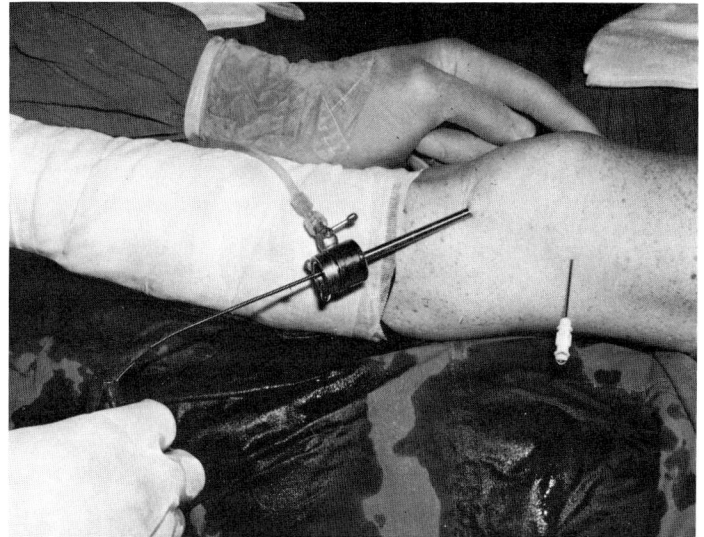

Fig. 4.1 Taking a specimen of synovium for histological study using micro-laryngeal cup forceps passed along the sheath of the arthroscope. The index of the left hand is used to apply counter-pressure to introduce synovium into the jaws of the forceps

Synovial biopsy

Synovial biopsy specimens may be obtained by three different methods.

'Blind' synovial biopsy

If no operating arthroscopic is available, good specimens of synovium can be obtained with a pair of cup or basket forceps small enough to be passed along the sheath of the arthroscope (Fig. 4.1). Although there is much to be said for a full examination of the knee as described in Chapter 2 in every patient, synovial biopsy is of greatest interest to rheumatologists who may wish to simplify the procedure by inserting the arthroscope from the lateral suprapatellar route and limiting the examination to the suprapatellar pouch alone. When a representative area of synovium has been identified, the tip of the instrument is brought close to the target and held still while the telescope is removed. Still holding the instruments immobile, biopsy forceps are passed along the sheath and the specimen removed. The joint is then irrigated thoroughly and the wound closed.

Although this technique does not allow the specimen to be taken under direct arthroscopic control, there is the advantage that large biopsy forceps can be used and a good volume of high quality tissue obtained. The technique is comparatively safe and uncomplicated but only one, or at the most two, specimens should be taken from the same site since repeated biopsy of the same area will result in penetration of both synovium and capsule, and

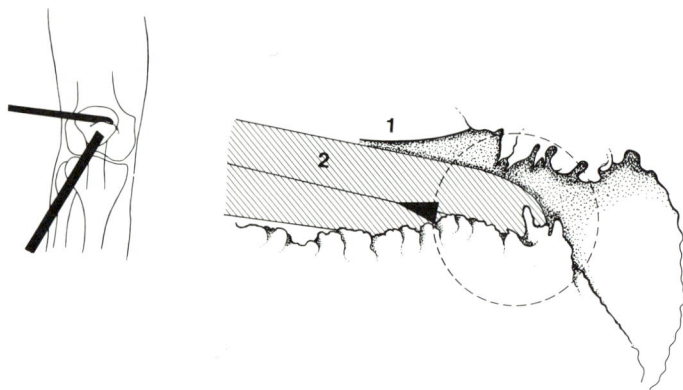

Fig. 4.2 Synovial biopsy by the double puncture technique using pituitary rongeurs (2) inserted from the lateral suprapatellar approach; (1) under-surface of the patella

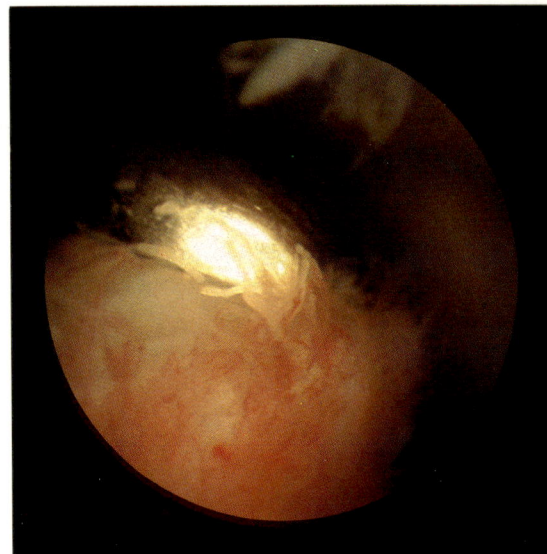

eventually of muscle and subcutaneous fat. Apart from the unnecessary trauma to the soft tissues caused by such a mishap, histological reports on tissues other than synovium are embarrassing to the surgeon and unhelpful to the patient.

Biopsy by double puncture

Synovial specimens can also be obtained from the suprapatellar pouch, after a full examination of the knee from the antero-lateral approach, with biopsy forceps passed along an instrument cannula inserted from the lateral suprapatellar route (Fig. 3.20). The best point of insertion of the instruments is determined by manipulation of the irrigation needle in the pouch. If the needle can reach the target easily, so will biopsy forceps inserted at the same point.

When the point of insertion has been selected, the instrument cannula should be inserted as described in Chapter 3, taking care not to damage either the articular cartilage of the patella or the arthroscope. With the knee straight, the biopsy forceps are identified through the arthroscope and a good specimen taken under direct arthroscopic control (Fig. 4.2). This technique yields the best specimens of tissue, partly because the larger telescope of the diagnostic arthroscope gives a better picture than the narrower telescope of the operating instruments and partly because good plump specimens of synovium can easily be obtained with the large biopsy forceps.

This technique also has the advantage that a representative sample of tissue can be identified under arthroscopic control, but there are the disadvantages that two incisions are needed and some expertise both with the arthroscope and with the operating instruments is required.

Biopsy using the operating arthroscope

Use of the operating arthroscope allows specimens to be taken under direct vision through one incision only. The knee is examined first with a diagnostic arthroscope and, once a suitable area of synovium has been identified, the operating instruments inserted. The biopsy forceps and narrow telescopes supplied with some diagnostic arthroscopes are quite adequate for this procedure, and can be inserted in place of the bridge on the diagnostic instruments (Fig. 3.1). A Wolf operating arthroscope can also be used but it offers no advantages over the simpler instruments for this procedure and requires a very slightly larger incision.

Although an operating arthroscope of any kind makes it easy to take synovial specimens under direct vision through only one incision, vision and orientation with the narrower telescope are more difficult than with the large diagnostic arthroscope and the biopsy specimens, which are only 1–2 mm in diameter, may show the histological appearances of surgical trauma more clearly than those of the underlying pathology. However much care is taken in the cleaning and maintenance of the biopsy forceps, specks of oil and debris may still contaminate the specimen and complicate the task of the pathologist unnecessarily.

Despite some disadvantages, the use of biopsy forceps in place of the bridge on a diagnostic arthroscope inserted from the lateral suprapatellar approach under local anaesthesia is probably the technique of choice for rheumatologists who require nothing more than a good view of inflamed synovium and a decent specimen for histological study.

Synovectomy

Plaques of pathological synovium can be excised completely without arthrotomy, but lesions suitable for this procedure are rare. Localised areas of synovial chondromatosis or pigmented synovitis 1–2 cm in diameter are sometimes seen, and can be removed with punch forceps and sharp dissection with scissors along the margin of the lesion. Such a procedure is more extensive than a biopsy, and can be described as a partial synovectomy.

With greater success in the control of acute rheumatoid arthritis by conservative means, the need to perform a synovectomy for this condition has diminished considerably, but if a chronic synovitis cannot be controlled adequately without operation anterior synovectomy can be performed using a standard powered shaver (Fig. 4.3). A powered instrument with a reciprocating blade has also been developed specifically for this procedure and is reported to be most effective, but is not yet generally available. To perform a synovectomy the shaver should be introduced from the lateral suprapatellar route and used to remove as much exuberant synovium as can be reached, taking care that only synovium is removed and not capsule or subcutaneous fat. Exuberant synovium can also be removed from the medial or lateral gutters and the intercondylar notch using pituitary rongeurs, and a technique for performing synovectomy with an electric resectoscope has recently been described (Aritomi H and Yamamoto M 1979). There is no evidence to suggest that the use of an electric resectoscope has any advantages over the existing powered instruments.

Although a synovectomy performed arthroscopically may not be as complete or as precise as a synovectomy performed through a wide arthrotomy, the period of rehabilitation is so much shorter and less uncomfortable after the arthroscopic procedure that it is greatly preferred by patients.

When a defect 1 or 2 cm in diameter is created in the synovium, the irrigating saline will quickly distend the subcutaneous tissues (Fig. 3.20) whichever technique is used and the procedure should therefore be planned carefully and completed swiftly once the synovium has been breached.

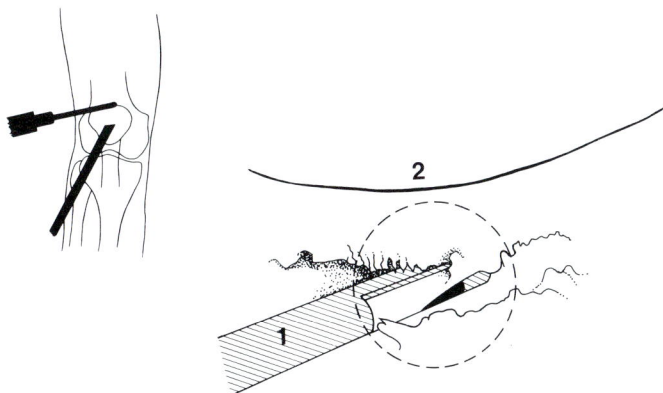

Fig. 4.3 Performing a synovectomy using the Stryker powered shaver (1) Patella (2)

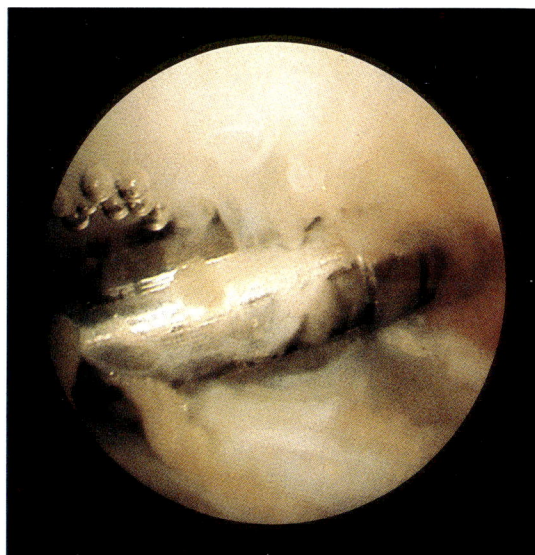

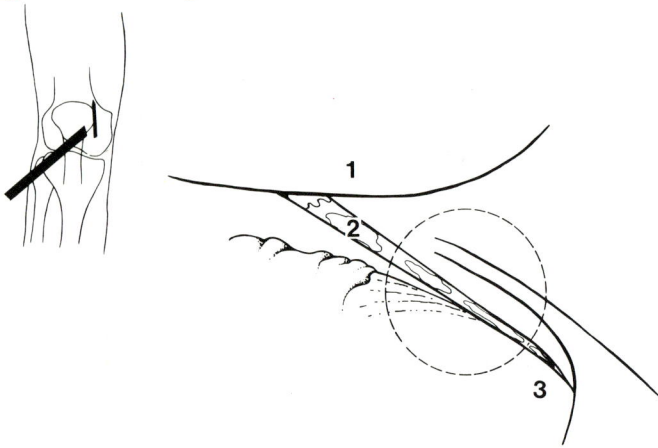

Fig. 4.4 Adhesion (2) between the medial femoral condyle (3) and the synovium of the suprapatellar pouch made tense by flexion of the knee (1) patella

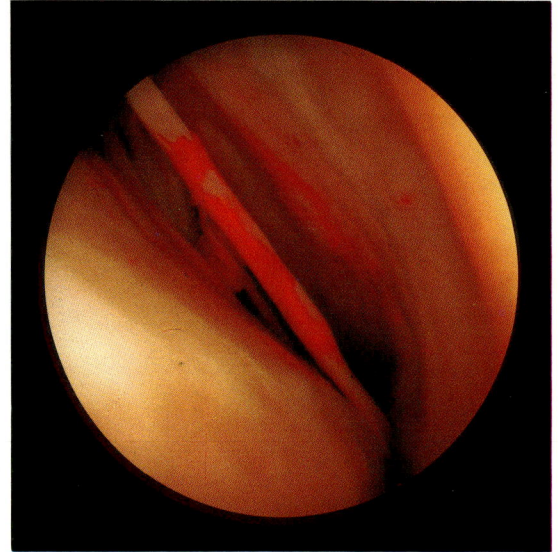

Adhesions and ankylosis

There is no doubt that fibrous adhesions can form between adjacent layers of synovium and between synovium and articular cartilage but the relationship of a patient's symptoms to these adhesions is not so clear. From a consideration of first principles, adhesions are likely to become taut during movement of the knee and to pull on the synovium as the knee is flexed or extended (Fig. 4.4). The arthrotomy needed for an open meniscectomy is sometimes followed by adhesions between the synovium and the femoral condyle and these adhesions can be seen to pucker the synovium on extreme flexion of the knee, but it is remarkable how seldom such adhesions give rise to serious problems.

Arthroscopy of the knee that has previously undergone arthrotomy is often made difficult by scarring and adhesions in the suprapatellar pouch and the medial or lateral gutters may be obliterated. Isolated adhesions encountered unexpectedly in the course of a routine arthroscopy can be ruptured by distension of the knee, broken with the arthroscopic sheath and obturator, divided through a second puncture, or cut with the operating arthroscope but adhesions which do not restrict flexion and can either be broken easily or divided with the delicate instruments of the operating arthroscope are unlikely to be the cause of important clinical symptoms. Although the results of dividing these adhesions is unpredictable and often disappointing, the procedure is simple and sometimes

followed by remarkable relief of pain, and is therefore worth doing.

In contrast to the disappointing results that may follow the division of thin adhesions in a joint that has a full range of movement, division of thicker adhesions can be most rewarding in joints with limited flexion. The best results are obtained in patients whose suprapatellar pouch has been obliterated by trauma to the lower end of the femur, infection of the joint or as a sequel to arthrotomy, and can be so successful that some patients originally admitted for a formal quadricepsplasty are able to return home on the day after operation with a greatly improved range of flexion after simple division of adhesions in the suprapatellar pouch.

Arthroscopic release of adhesions does not replace physiotherapy as the mainstay of treatment for post-traumatic knee stiffness. Vigorous mobilisation of the knee after femoral fractures is still needed, and operation should not even be considered until the fracture is soundly united and all improvement from physiotherapy has ceased. If these requirements are met arthroscopic division of the adhesions is indicated, so that stiffness of the knee becomes an indication for arthroscopy rather than a contra-indication.

Division of adhesions

The procedure begins with a careful examination under general anaesthesia to assess movement once pain and reflex muscle spasm have been abolished, and the knee flexed fully to break down the weaker adhesions. Because adhesions are usually vascular, inflation of the tourniquet before arthroscopy is strongly recommended.

A few adhesions may rupture as the joint is distended with saline to produce a 'popping' sensation under the surgeon's fingers, and greater pressure can be applied to the saline by squeezing the irrigation reservoir to rupture more adhesions. Some indication of the extent of the adhesions can be gauged by noting the volume of saline that the knee will accommodate. The normal knee will hold 60–80 ml of saline, but an ankylosed knee may be fully distended after the injection of only 5–10 ml. After distension of the knee, the arthroscope should be inserted and the joint examined in the usual way, taking particular care not to bend the arthroscope by injudicious attempts to break adhesions by using it as a crow-bar.

Detailed examination of the joint will probably be made impossible by adhesions obstructing the free passage of the arthroscope in the suprapatellar pouch and the medial and lateral gutters. Once a general impression of the distribution of the adhesions has been obtained, the straight knife or scissors can be inserted from the lateral suprapatellar approach and the adhesions divided under arthroscopic control. The delicate cutting instruments of the operating arthroscope have little place in this procedure, for which the strongest and sharpest cutting instruments are preferable. When the arthroscope can be moved freely throughout both the suprapatellar pouch and the lateral gutter, the arthroscope and operating instruments may be withdrawn and the joint irrigated thoroughly with saline before releasing the tourniquet.

Release of ankylosis

Adhesions are sometimes so dense that the synovial cavity is completely obliterated and insertion of the arthroscope from the anterolateral route proves impossible. This difficulty may arise after infection or major trauma, and occasionally after total knee replacement with a surface replacement prosthesis when insertion of a sharp trocar from the antero-lateral approach is particularly undesirable because of the risk of damage to the smooth surface of the prosthesis. This difficulty can be overcome if, instead of inserting the arthroscope from the antero-lateral route, the trocar and cannula of the operating

instruments are first inserted from the lateral suprapatellar approach. When it has been established that the trocar lies in the obliterated pouch, it can be used to rupture adhesions in the pouch and the lateral gutter. While manipulation of the trocar alone will not create enough space to restore flexion, the space created is usually large enough to admit the arthroscope for a preliminary examination. The pouch can then be developed fully with a knife taking great care to ensure that the tip of the knife remains in the suprapatellar pouch, and the adhesions are divided until the knife blade moves freely, irrigating the joint frequently (Fig. 4.5). When the pouch and lateral gutter have been freed, the trocar and cannula can be inserted from the antero-lateral route, and the adhesions lying in front of the femur divided. If a gentle manipulation does not then restore movement after division of these adhesions, the medial gutter should be developed with instruments inserted through a third incision at the medial edge of the medial femoral condyle, about 1 cm above the level of the tibial plateau.

The release of a dense fibrous ankylosis will produce a large quantity of fibrous debris which must be removed from the joint. A powered shaver will serve as a 'vacuum cleaner' for this purpose, but the debris can be removed just as quickly and effectively, and much more cheaply, with a large sucker or a pair of forceps.

When all the adhesions in the anterior compartments of the knee have been divided, the operating instruments can be inserted from the postero-medial approach. The postero-medial compartment can be difficult to enter if strong adhesions are present and this approach should not be attempted unless the surgeon is able to perform a posteromedial insertion in the normal knee with complete confidence. Once entered, any adhesions in the postero-medial compartment can be broken down with the trocar or divided with a knife. Surprisingly, the release of these posterior adhesions seldom results in any noticeable improvement in the range of flexion or extension.

When all accessible adhesions have been cut the joint is irrigated thoroughly and re-examined completely, the tourniquet released and the joint again irrigated until all blood has been cleared. The improvement in the range of flexion is then measured, a firm wool and crepe dressing applied and physiotherapy commenced, preferably in the Recovery Room.

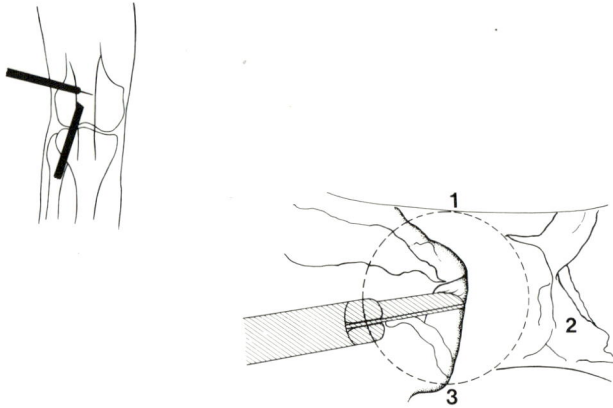

Fig. 4.5 Release of a dense fibrous ankylosis of the suprapatellar pouch using a knife inserted from the lateral suprapatellar route. (1) Under-surface of the patella; (2) dense fibrous adhesions in suprapatellar pouch; (3) anterior surface of the femur

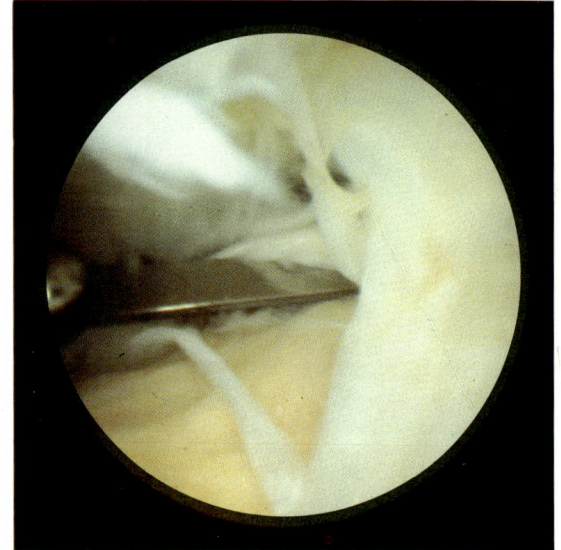

An immediate improvement of 20° to 30° is usual after this procedure, but the improvement in the patient's symptoms is by no means proportional to the improvement in the range of movement and it is not unknown for the patient to report a dramatic improvement in the symptoms after a disappointingly small increase in the range of flexion. Physiotherapy should be continued as an out-patient, and may be rewarded with a further improvement in the range of movement.

If the symptoms persist a second procedure may be more successful. It is a tribute to the atraumatic nature of arthroscopic surgery that patients are willing to undergo this procedure for a second time.

Synovial shelf excision

The synovial folds of the knee have already been described in Chapter 2. The classification of these folds has proved difficult and has been bedevilled by the Dog-Latin aliases mentioned on pp. 14, 15 and 16 (Fig. 2.13). The medial synovial shelf lies in the coronal plane and arises in the fat pad below the lower pole of the patella to run proximally for a variable distance, sometimes extending above the medial patellar plica, which it usually crosses at a right angle. The 'shelf' is so named from its arthroscopic appearance which is that of a pale, sharp-edged membrane that lies in the horizontal plane during arthroscopy.

Although first described in 1939 by Iino, the medial synovial shelf was not widely recognised until arthro-scopy became a routine procedure and examination of the distended synovial cavity under magnification from within led to the recognition of folds or shelves of synovium not readily noticeable in an empty joint that has been sliced open either post-mortem or at operation. The medial synovial shelf should not be confused with the medial suprapatellar plica, which lies above the patella in the horizontal plane and may extend right across the joint to divide it into two almost separate compartments. The plica does not appear to have any great clinical significance apart from affording refuge for loose bodies and offering a convenient piece of tissue for synovial biopsy.

The medial synovial shelf is a normal structure that is more obvious in some patients than others, and is absent altogether in approximately 20 per cent of patients. The shelf can often be felt as a tender ridge crossing the medial femoral condyle, but must be distinguished from the synovium of the medial gutter. The shelf is usually swollen and tender when there is generalised synovitis in the rest of the joint, and is then seen as a thickened and inflamed fold instead of a thin crescentic shelf. The shelf sweeps across the medial femoral condyle during flexion of the knee, and comes into contact with the area of femoral condyle that strikes the anterior horn of the meniscus in full extension. If the 'impingement lesion' is present (Figs. 2.18, 2.19), the shelf will be seen to sweep across it in approximately 45° of flexion, which often corresponds with the position in which the patient's knee is most painful. The 'impingement lesion' and the groove in the medial femoral condyle described by Patel (1978) may be one and the same.

Synovial shelf syndrome

As every clinician dealing with knee disorders will be only too acutely aware, many patients, especially adolescent girls, suffer pain around the patella when the knee is flexed. Such patients are often said to be suffering from 'chondromalacia patellae' but the arthroscopist will often find this explanation unsatisfactory because he knows that many patients with this diagnosis have a patella that is arthroscopically normal, while many others with gross irregularities of the articular cartilage of the patella have no symptoms whatever that can be attributed to the patello-femoral joint.

The synovial shelf syndrome, which has been well described by Fujisawa (1976) and Patel (1978), is characterised by pain on flexion of the knee, tenderness of the synovial shelf, and an absence of patello-femoral tenderness. A blow to the front of the knee, often a dashboard injury, is a common precipitating factor. The syndrome should be suspected in patients with anterior knee pain arising from the patello-femoral area who have no tenderness on pressure over the patella itself, but who have localised tenderness when the synovial shelf is rolled against the underlying medial femoral condyle. Some will also be found to have a distinct 'painful arc' from 45° to 60° of flexion corresponding with the movement of the synovial shelf across the femoral condyle, and it is easy to speculate that contact between an inflamed or scarred synovial shelf and the femoral condyle could be the cause of this discomfort. Although the synovial shelf syndrome usually affects the medial side, symptoms may also arise from damage to the lateral synovial shelf and can also be relieved by arthroscopic excision of the offending structure.

The results of excision of the synovial shelf are encouraging. Several studies have shown that approximately 80 per cent of patients with pain on flexion of the knee, a history of injury, a broad synovial shelf and tenderness medial to the patella without any other abnormality on clinical or radiological examination can expect to be relieved of their symptoms by arthroscopic excision of the synovial shelf. Some cynics have observed that many open operations for 'chondromalacia patellae' and pain on the medial side of the knee in young patients result in either division of the synovial shelf or a relaxation of the medial parapatellar tissues, including the shelf, and suggest that lateral release, tibial tubercle transposition, exploratory arthrotomy, medial meniscectomy and even patellectomy may be little more than complicated techniques for dividing or relaxing the medial synovial shelf. Rival cynics have asked why this condition has reached epidemic proportions in certain centres during the last few years and find difficulty in understanding why the synovial shelf syndrome did not afflict the human race until the arthroscope was invented. This problem is unresolved at the time of writing, but it does seem likely that the medial and lateral synovial shelf syndromes exist, that the symptoms can be relieved dramatically by arthroscopic excision of the shelf, and that the diagnosis is made far too often.

Whatever the explanation, there can be no doubt either that the reported results of excision of the shelf are comparable with those of more drastic procedures, or that the operation is less traumatic. Arthroscopic excision of the synovial shelf is a simple procedure that can be performed either by the double or single puncture techniques and it is this very simplicity which has made the medial synovial shelf syndrome such a seductive diagnosis for the arthroscopic surgeon.

Excision of the shelf with the operating arthroscope

The aim of operation should be the excision of a segment of the distal third of the shelf at least 1 cm in length and extending the full depth of the shelf, and not just simple division of the shelf. Simple division of the shelf alone can result in the development of a band of dense fibrous tissue in the place of the shelf and a recurrence of the symptoms (Fig. 4.6). Histological study of the synovial tissue from these lesions shows the appearances of chronic synovitis with hyaline change.

The shelf can be excised with the instruments of the operating arthroscope inserted from the antero-lateral route, with the knee held straight (Fig. 3.4). Two incisions in the shelf are made with the operating scissors, at least 1 cm apart and extending into normal synovium. The irrigating saline will dissect a tissue plane below the shelf, which can then be excised neatly by connecting the two incisions with scissors and removing the segment of shelf with basket forceps

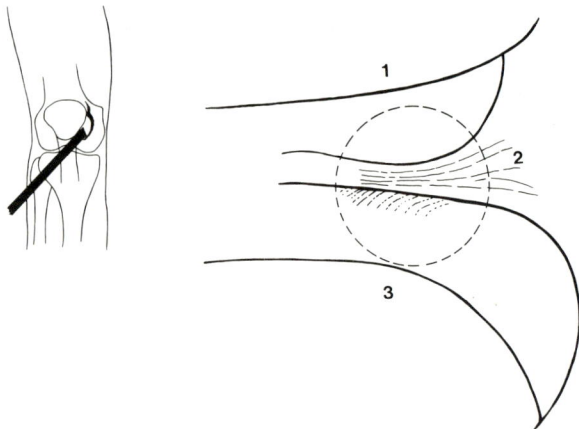

Fig. 4.6 A band of dense fibrous tissue (2) which had formed at the site of an earlier excision of the medial synovial shelf; (1) patella (3) medial femoral condyle

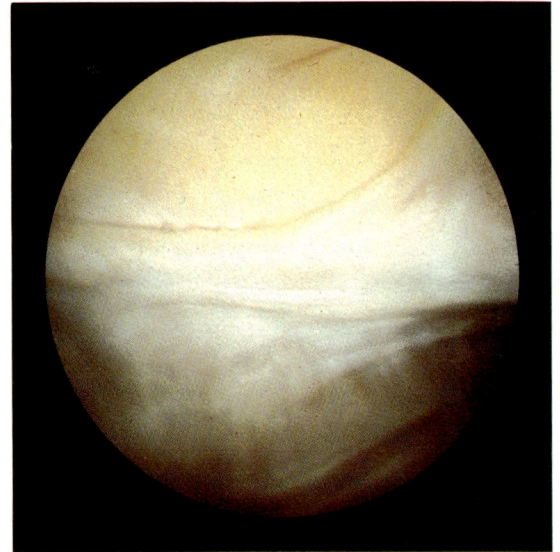

(Fig. 4.7). If an impingement lesion is present on the femoral condyle, this can also be trimmed with the basket forceps.

Wide excision of the medial shelf can be accomplished most easily by applying gentle traction to the lateral end of the shelf with a pair of grasping forceps inserted from the lateral suprapatellar route while the base of the shelf is divided with the scissors of an operating arthroscope inserted from the antero-lateral route (Fig. 4.8). This technique allows the whole of

the shelf to be excised simply and effectively (Fig. 4.9) but requires some expertise with the operating arthroscope.

Excision of the shelf by double puncture

Wide excision of the medial shelf can also be accomplished with cup forceps or rongeurs inserted from the lateral suprapatellar approach, but this technique has the disadvantage that in some patients the anatomy of the patello-femoral joint is such that

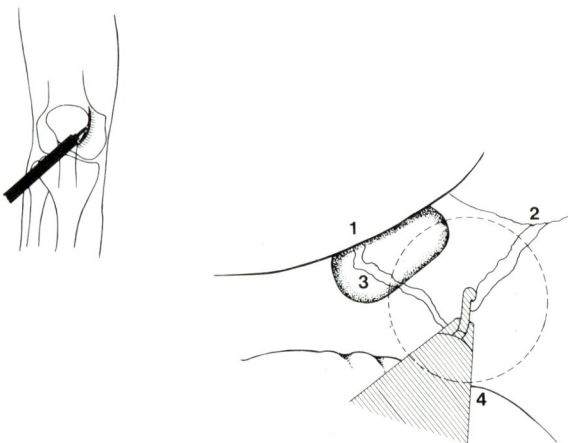

Fig. 4.7 Excision of synovial shelf using a Wolf operating arthroscope. (1) Patella (2) cut edge of synovium (3) air bubble (4) anterior surface of femur

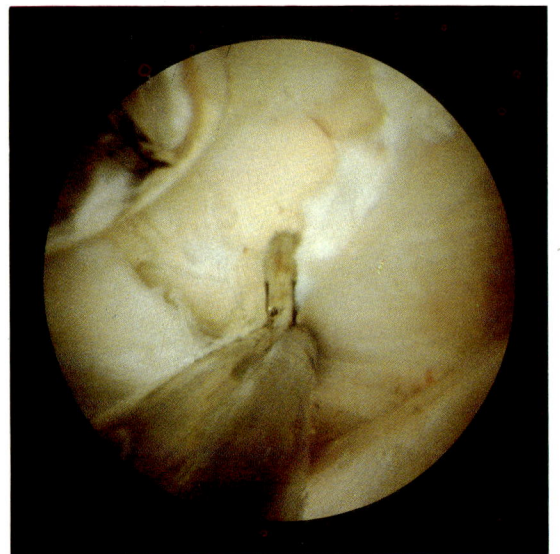

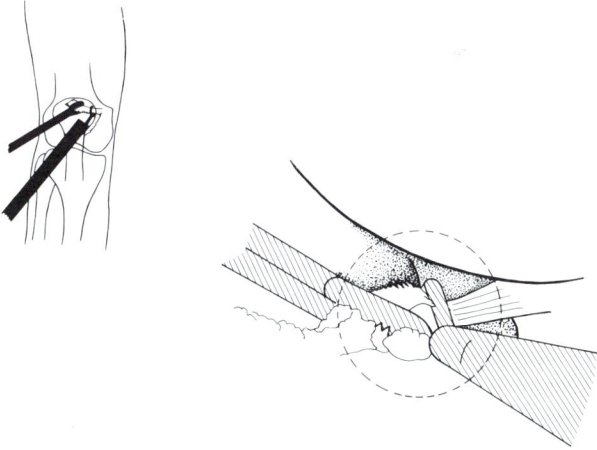

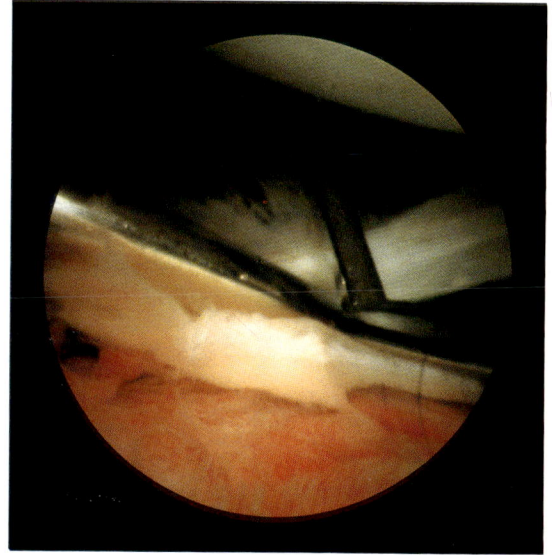

Fig. 4.8 Excising the medial synovial shelf using the scissors of the operating arthroscope while applying traction to the shelf with tendon tunnelling forceps

the shelf cannot be reached with instruments inserted from this route. This problem is not uncommon in men, whose intercondylar notch may be deeper than those of women with a corresponding prominence of the central facet of the patella. Because of this difficulty, it is essential before inserting the instruments from the lateral suprapatellar approach for this procedure to be quite certain that the tip of the irrigation needle can be made to touch the shelf with ease. If this can be done, the needle is withdrawn and the operating instruments inserted at the same point with full confidence that access to the shelf will be uncomplicated. If the shelf cannot be touched with the irrigation needle, either the single puncture technique should be used or the arthroscope moved to the lateral suprapatellar approach and the instruments

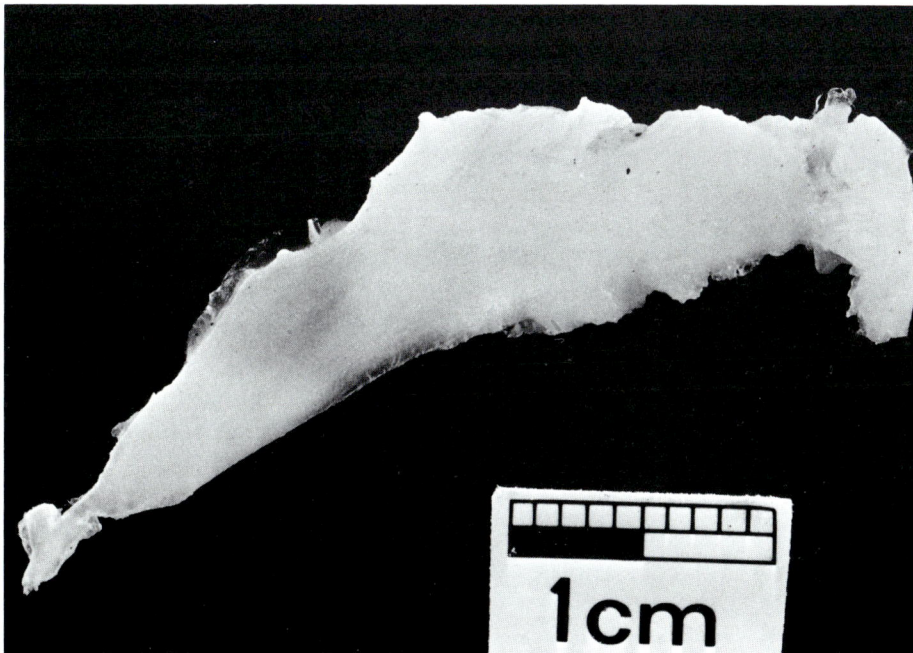

Fig. 4.9 A shelf excised arthroscopically using the technique illustrated in Figure 4.8

to the antero-lateral. With this arrangement of instruments and with the knee held straight, the shelf can be removed quickly and easily with either straight or curved rongeurs.

Aftercare

After excision of medial or lateral shelves, the wounds should be closed with one stitch each and the usual wool and crepe dressing applied. As with other arthroscopic procedures, straight leg raising is almost always possible on recovery from the anaesthetic, with flexion to 90° within 24 hours of operation. Most patients experience some discomfort at the site of the shelf resection for 2–3 weeks, and the symptoms may persist for 6–8 weeks after operation before settling completely. Some synovitis is inevitable after this procedure, but can be minimised by the administration of an anti-inflammatory drug such as ketoprofen 50 mg three times daily for 10 days.

Lateral retinacular release

Lateral release of the extensor mechanism is an established open operation for 'chondromalacia patellae' or subluxation of the patella but can also be performed arthroscopically. The incision in the capsule should extend from the insertion of the patellar tendon to a point 4 cm (1½″) above the upper pole of the patella and should include the patellar insertion of vastus lateralis (Fig. 4.10), but the skin,

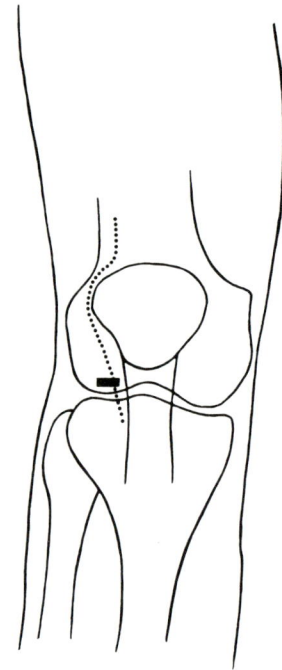

Fig. 4.10 The line of capsular incision for lateral release of the extensor mechanism

subcutaneous tissues and synovium need not be divided. The exact indications for the procedure have yet to be defined precisely, but at present include subluxation of the patella, abnormal lateral tracking of the patella with more than one quarter of the patella overhanging the lateral margin of the femur in extension (Fig. 4.11), and chondral defects in the patellar surface.

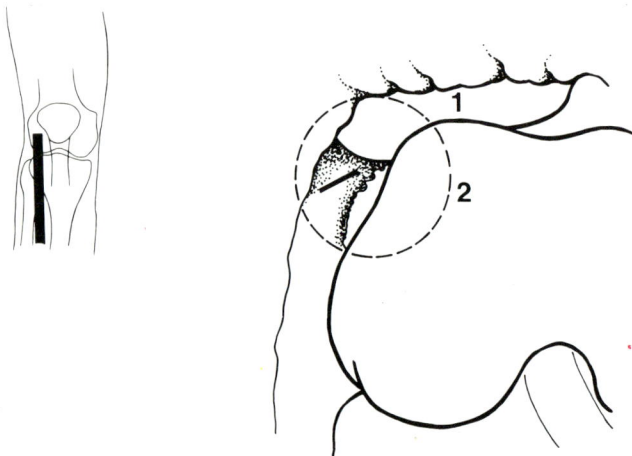

Fig. 4.11 Lateral tracking of the patella with the lateral edge of the patella (1) overhanging the edge of the lateral femoral condyle (2) seen from the lateral gutter

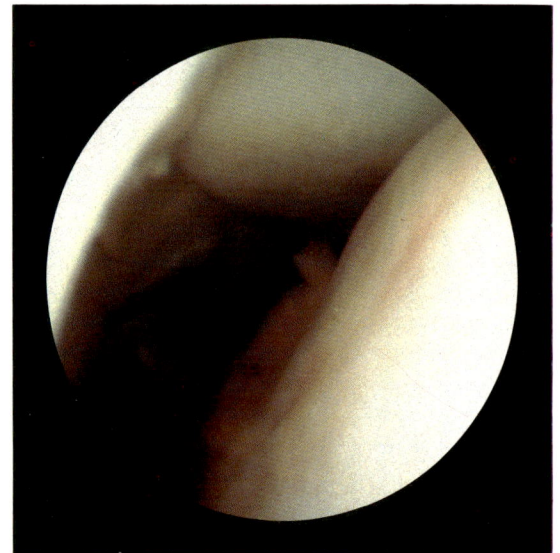

Technique

There are at least three ways in which a lateral release can be performed arthroscopically. Whichever technique is used, it is advisable to infiltrate the line of capsular incision with bupivacaine 0.5 per cent containing adrenaline to reduce post-operative pain and minimise bleeding from the superior branch of the lateral geniculate artery, which is inevitably divided if the procedure is performed correctly. Some surgeons prefer to incise synovium as well as capsule, but there is as yet no evidence to determine whether this is necessary or not.

1. The simplest technique is to pass a Smillie knife through the incision used for insertion of the arthroscope from the antero-lateral route and to direct it proximally. The 'V' of the blade should be placed carefully over the capsule, which can then be divided as far as necessary both proximally and distally taking special care to curve the incision over the supero-lateral angle of the patella (Fig. 4.12). Observation of the passage of the knife with the arthroscope from the antero-medial or suprapatellar approach is difficult and unhelpful, and the criticism is sometimes made that lateral release performed in this way is a 'blind' rather than an arthroscopic procedure.

2. The criticism that the procedure is blind rather than arthroscopic can be overcome by dividing both synovium and capsule with a long handled knife inserted from the medial suprapatellar approach and manipulated under arthroscopic control from the antero-lateral approach. The point of insertion of the knife makes it necessary to divide the capsule rather lower than most surgeons would choose, and impossible to curve the line of capsular incision over the supero-lateral corner of the patella to divide the stout attachment of vastus lateralis. This technique is not recommended.

3. A combination of blind and arthroscopic technique has been developed by Dr R Metcalf. A pair of Metzenbaum scissors is introduced at the point of insertion of the arthroscope from the antero-lateral route and used to develop a subcutaneous tissue plane as far as the lateral edge of the patella. A second skin incision is then made over the tips of the scissors and the subcutaneous tissue plane extended medially in front of the patellar tendon. The distal portion of the synovium capsule is then divided with the Metzenbaum scissors, and the proximal portion with the scissors of the operating arthroscope.

As with synovial biopsy or partial synovectomy, the irrigating saline will track through the synovial defect and produce a boggy swelling in the subcutaneous tissues that can be expected to settle completely within 24 hours.

Aftercare

When the release is complete, the tourniquet is released and the joint irrigated in the usual way. A pad of rolled gauze, wool or foam is applied to the full length of the capsular incision and held in place with

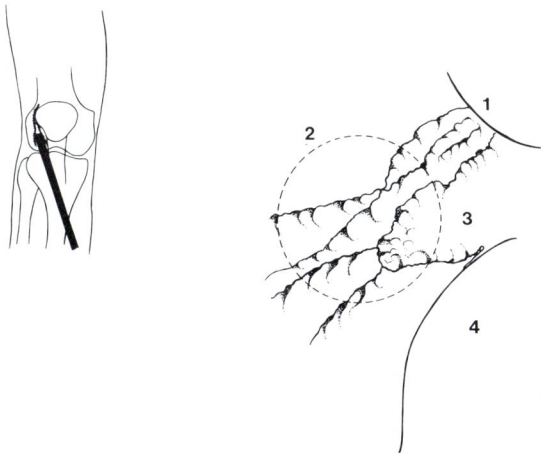

Fig. 4.12 Arthroscopic view of the line of lateral release of the synovium and capsule (1) patella (2) synovium (3) cut edge of capsule (4) lateral femoral condyle

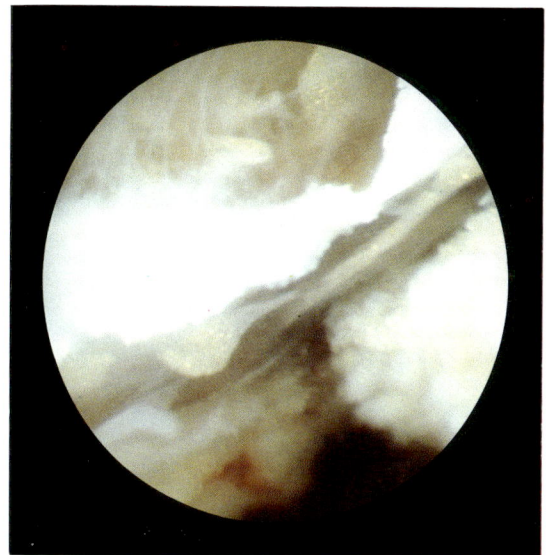

a dressing of orthopaedic wool and a crepe bandage. The area to which the pad should be applied can be marked with ink as suggested by Dr R Metcalf so that it can be reapplied correctly by the patient if the bandage should slip. These precautions are necessary to minimise the risk of haematoma formation, which is painful and can lead to infection. Active physiotherapy, including flexion, is instituted at once. Some discomfort at the site of the capsular division is usual and may persist for five to six weeks.

Excision of fat-pad

Inflammation of pads of fat and synovial fronds have been incriminated as a cause of anterior knee pain since at least 1904 (Hoffa 1904) but the condition has sometimes been considered a diagnosis of desperation. Whether swollen fat-pads cause genuine symptoms or not, there are times when a patient with pain or tenderness around the patellar tendon, made worse by extension of the knee, is found to have a particularly large and succulent fat-pad which can be removed arthroscopically with the relief of symptoms. Whatever the relationship of the patient's symptoms to the fat-pad, there is no doubt that it is a source of great irritation to the arthroscopist when it falls over the lens of the arthroscope and blocks vision. Even when this does not occur, its size and shape is difficult to assess from the antero-lateral, antero-medial, or central approaches because it lies so close to the lens.

It is possible to remove the fat-pad with rongeurs inserted from the antero-medial route but the jaws of the instrument come to lie so close to an arthroscope inserted from the antero-lateral or central approach that control of the instrument is difficult. The procedure is made easier if the arthroscope is transferred to the lateral suprapatellar approach, and the fat-pad removed piece-meal with a combination of straight and curved rongeurs inserted from the antero-lateral or antero-medial approach (Fig. 4.13).

If the surgeon possesses a powered shaver, it can be used to remove the fat-pad when it is considered to be the cause of symptoms, or even when it obscures the arthroscopic view. The removal of healthy tissue simply because it makes life difficult for the surgeon by interfering with the view down the arthroscope is not in keeping with the atraumatic spirit of arthroscopic surgery. If the surgeon cannot see everything he wishes down the arthroscope, it is the author's opinion that he should concentrate on improving his arthroscopic technique rather than disguise his deficiencies by taking a powered tool to normal tissue.

Lipomata and synoviomata—Pedunculated tumours arising from the synovium of the medial or lateral gutters are sometimes seen, and may cause symptoms very similar to those associated with a meniscus injury or a loose body. These tumours can be removed neatly by avulsing them with a pair of pituitary rongeurs applied to their base (Fig. 4.14) leaving a small defect in the synovium (Fig. 4.15).

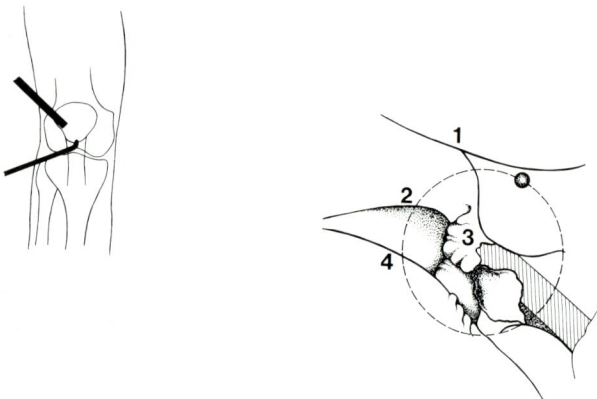

Fig. 4.13 Removing a hypertrophic fat-pad (3) with instruments inserted from the antero-lateral route and seen from the lateral suprapatellar approach (1) patella (2) medial synovial shelf (4) femur

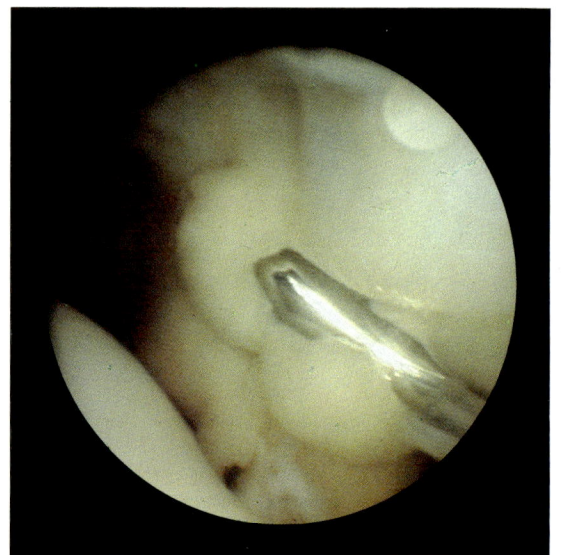

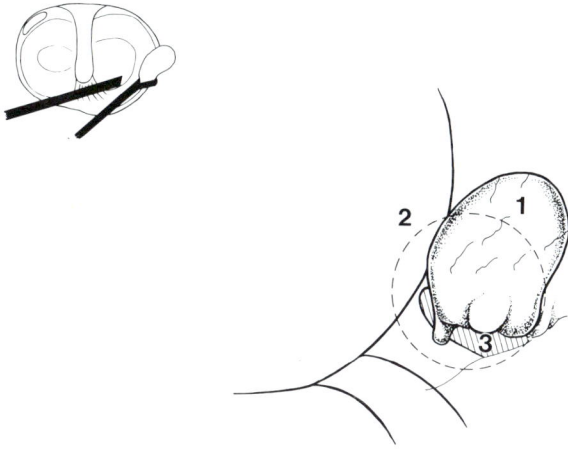

Fig. 4.14 A pedunculated benign synovioma (1) in the medial gutter grasped at its base with curved rongeurs (3) (2) medial femoral condyle

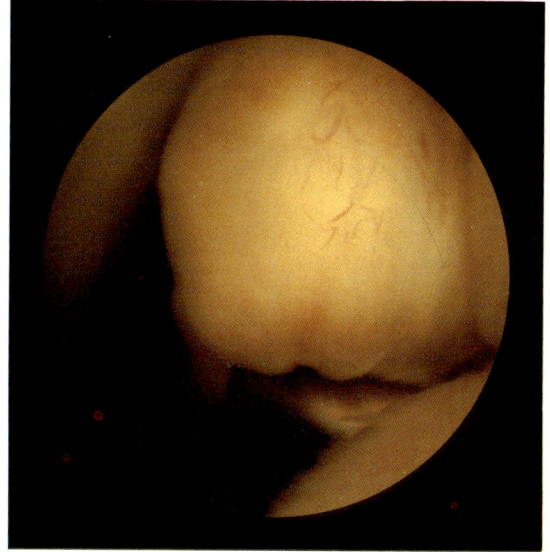

If the pedicle cannot be identified precisely, which is a problem if the tumour is particularly large, a short incision can be made over the tumour so that it can be lifted out of the knee and divided at its base under direct vision. Histological study of such lesions usually shows them to be either a lipoma or a benign synovioma.

Crystal synovitis

Although irrigation of the joint can scarcely be considered an arthroscopic operation, the pain and effusion of crystal-induced synovitis is almost always relieved dramatically by simple joint irrigation and such relief can last for many months. Symptoms of other types of synovitis, including that associated with osteoarthrosis, may also be relieved by irrigation.

It is not known whether this relief of pain is due to the removal of abnormal synovial fluid and joint debris, lavage of the synovium, temporary hypothermia of the synovium from irrigation with cold saline, or to some metabolic alteration induced by contact

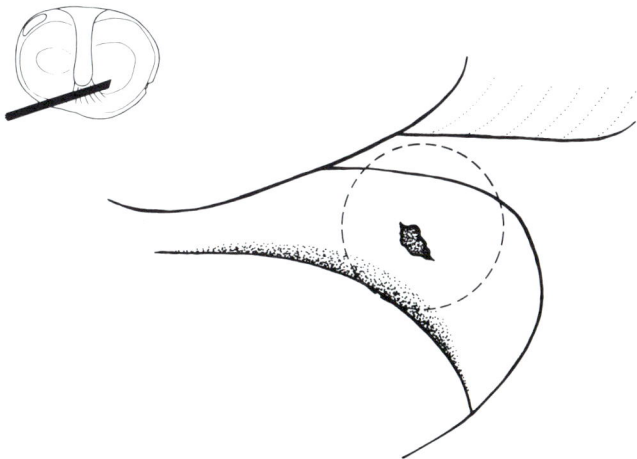

Fig. 4.15 The site of attachment of the synovioma illustrated in Figure 4.14 after it had been avulsed

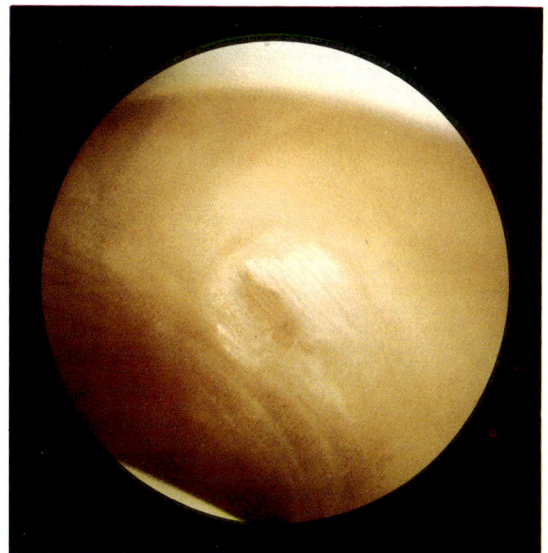

with irrigation fluid. The fact that we cannot explain the mechanism of this pain relief is taken by some as proof that it does not exist and by others as proof of our ignorance.

REFERENCES

Aritomi H, Yamamoto M 1979 A Method of Arthroscopic Surgery. Clinical Evaluation of Synovectomy with the Electric Resectoscope and Removal of Loose Bodies in the Knee Joint. Orthopedic Clinics of North America 10: 565–584

Fujisawa Y 1976 Problems caused by the Medial and Lateral synovial folds of the Patella. Kansetsukyo 1: 40–44

Hoffa A 1904 The influence of the adipose tissue with regard to the pathology of the knee joint. Journal of the American Medical Association 43: 795–796

Iino S 1939 Normal Arthroscopic Findings in the knee joint in adult cadavers. Journal of the Japanese Orthopaedic Association 14: 467, 523

Patel D 1978 Arthroscopy of the plicae-synovial folds and their significance. The American Journal of Sports Medicine 6: 217–225

5

Loose bodies, foreign bodies, joint surfaces and ligaments

Loose bodies

The presence of a loose body is usually apparent from the clinical history, examination and radiography. Arthroscopy is therefore of limited importance in assessment of the patient apart from confirming the diagnosis and evaluating the size, mobility and number of loose bodies present but is nevertheless useful in determining the true size of loose bodies that consist of a mass of cartilage surrounding a small nidus of bone or calcification, in discovering loose bodies that are not calcified, and in identifying the site from which the loose bodies arose. Careful inspection of the under-surface of the patella and femoral condyles will often reveal a defect that corresponds with the loose body, and experience of arthroscopy leads to the conclusion that osteochondral fractures are more common than is generally believed while idiopathic loose bodies and 'osteochondritis dissecans' are less common. The arthroscope is also helpful in the assessment of those isolated areas of calcification that occur along the joint margins and in the intercondylar notch, sometimes reported by radiologists as 'loose' bodies. Arthroscopy may demonstrate that these lesions are in fact covered by synovium and are so densely adherent to the surrounding tissue that excision is likely to be more difficult than anticipated.

Arthroscopic removal of loose bodies

The arthroscopic removal of loose bodies proceeds in three stages:

1. Finding the loose body,
2. Catching the loose body, and
3. Removing the loose body.

Finding the loose body. A plain radiograph before operation is helpful in locating the loose body but does not exclude the possibility of the loose body moving as the limb is prepared for operation. Arthroscopy has the advantages that the entire joint can be examined more thoroughly than at arthrotomy and the loose body can be pursued as it moves around the knee from one compartment to another. For these reasons, loose bodies are more easily found at arthroscopy than at arthrotomy.

The suprapatellar pouch is the first place to look. Special attention must be paid to the medial suprapatellar plica because it may conceal the loose body, particularly if the plica is large and divides the joint into two almost separate compartments. The telescope should be passed beyond the plica and the proximal recess of the suprapatellar pouch examined carefully (Fig. 5.1). While examining the suprapatellar pouch, the telescope should be turned upwards to examine the under-surface of the patella for any defects that might have been caused by an osteochondral fracture.

If no loose body has been found at this stage, the surgeon should pause before flexing the knee to enter the medial compartment. Loose bodies are denser than saline and sink to the bottom of a knee distended with saline so that those in the suprapatellar pouch will fall into the medial or lateral gutter while the suprapatellar pouch is examined and, when the knee is flexed, slip easily into the posterior compartment, from which retrieval is more difficult. The possibility of a loose body lying in one of the gutters must therefore be considered before the knee is flexed. Palpation through the skin from below upwards may identify a loose body which can be pushed back into

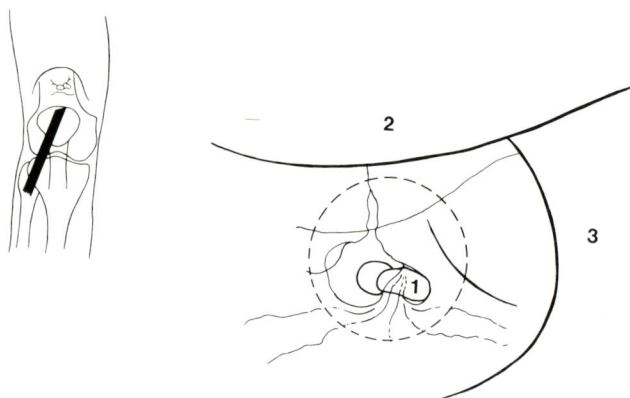

Fig. 5.1 Three loose bodies (1) concealed behind a fold of synovium at the apex of the suprapatellar pouch, above the medial suprapatellar plica (3)—(2) undersurface of patella

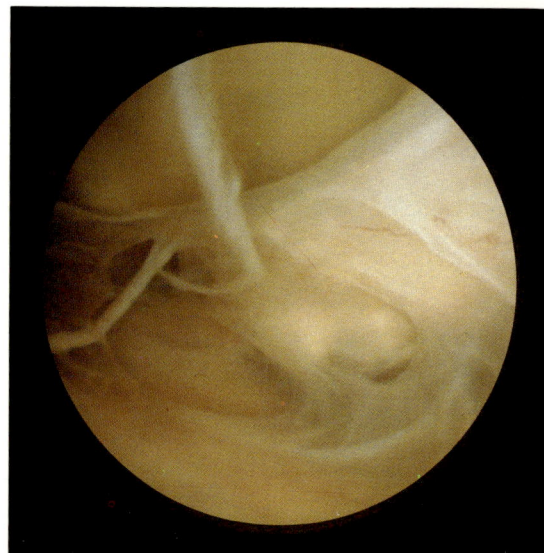

the pouch and held there for removal, but if this manoeuvre is unsuccessful, the normal routine examination of the knee described in Chapter 2 should be interrupted and the arthroscope slipped down into the lateral gutter to examine the popliteus tendon and the entrance to its tunnel, a favourite refuge for the smaller loose bodies. If the loose body has still not been found, it can only be in the back of the medial gutter, the intercondylar notch, or one of the posterior compartments.

The medial gutter should then be examined more thoroughly, taking the precaution of applying gentle pressure to the postero-medial jointline to block the route from the medial gutter to the postero-medial compartment. If the gutter is clear, the knee can be flexed safely and the medial compartment entered and examined in the usual way but with special attention to the anterior horn of the medial meniscus, which can also conceal small loose bodies.

The telescope is then passed across to the intercondylar notch. Large loose bodies become jammed in the intercondylar notch but small or flat bodies can skate away to the lateral compartment or, worse, to the postero-medial compartment. Loose bodies can only reach the posterior compartments from the back of the medial or lateral gutters or through the intercondylar notch, and care must be taken not to nudge the loose body into the postero-medial compartment with the tip of the telescope. The classical birthplace of osteochondritic fragments should also

be examined before leaving the notch to enter the lateral compartment.

In the lateral compartment special attention should be paid to possible defects in the articular surface of the femur and to the undersurface of the meniscus in its posterior third. Loose bodies, and sometimes foreign bodies, can elude discovery by slipping beneath the posterior horn of the meniscus but their presence is given way by a curiously stiff and elevated appearance of the posterior third of the meniscus which makes it easy to slip the arthroscope or rongeurs under the meniscus as described in Chapter 2 (Fig. 5.2 and Fig. 5.3).

If the loose body has still not been found, the postero-medial and postero-lateral compartments should be examined with 30° and 70° telescopes as described in Chapter 2, but if the postero-medial compartment cannot be entered from the antero-lateral approach a postero-medial insertion of the arthroscope will be needed and will usually reveal the loose body in the inferior recess of the postero-medial compartment. If the loose body is not in the postero-medial compartment, the lateral suprapatellar insertion can be used to examine the popliteus tunnel and the postero-lateral corner of the joint in detail by directing the arthroscope downwards into the lateral gutter with the knee extended.

If this routine has been followed correctly without finding a loose body, the surgeon should enlarge the lateral suprapatellar incision to approximately 2 cm,

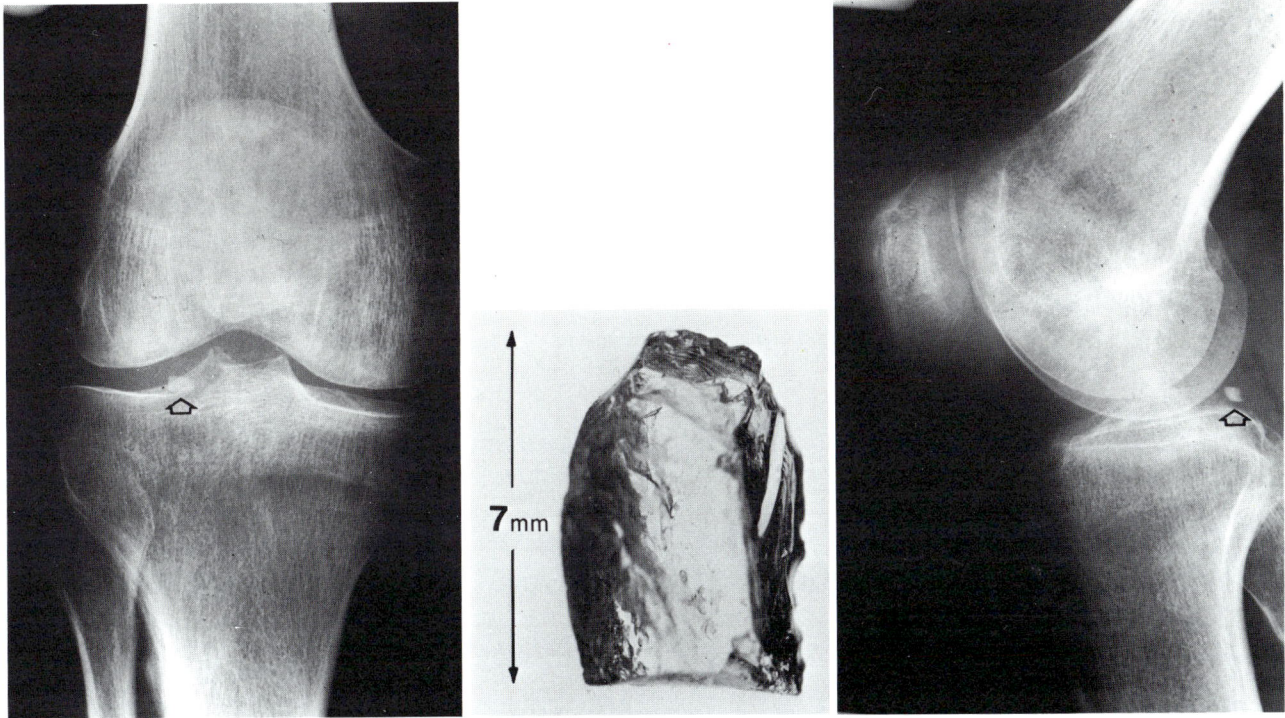

Fig. 5.2 A fragment of glass which had entered the knee anteriorly and come to rest beneath the posterior horn of the lateral meniscus. The fragment, shown in the centre, is clearly seen on both the anterior and lateral radiographs

change his gloves, and cautiously insert one sterile finger into the suprapatellar pouch to search for abnormal recesses of the suprapatellar pouch that might have escaped inspection with the arthroscope. However carefully the suprapatellar pouch is examined, there is always the possibility that there is an anomalous pouch of synovium large enough to conceal a loose body. In one such patient, a pouch of synovium was found arising from the supero-lateral corner of the knee and extending downwards and laterally beside the femur to lie deep to the ilio-tibial tract, making it impossible to palpate the loose body through

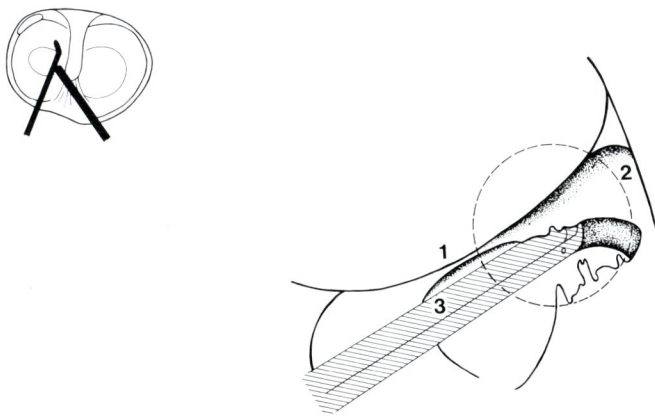

Fig. 5.3 Small angled rongeurs (3) passed beneath the posterior horn of the lateral meniscus (2) and seen from the antero-medial approach (1) lateral femoral condyle

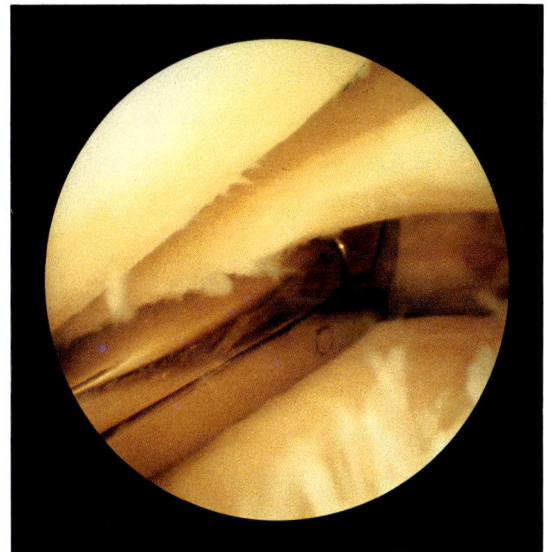

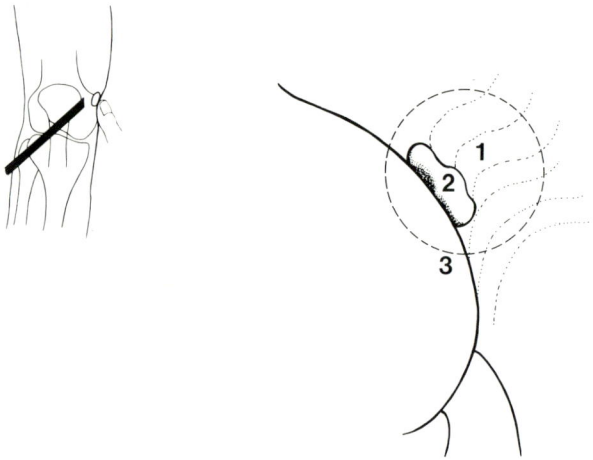

Fig. 5.4 A loose body (2) is prevented from slipping from the suprapatellar pouch into the medial gutter by external finger pressure applied to the medial wall of the knee (1)—(3) medial femoral condyle

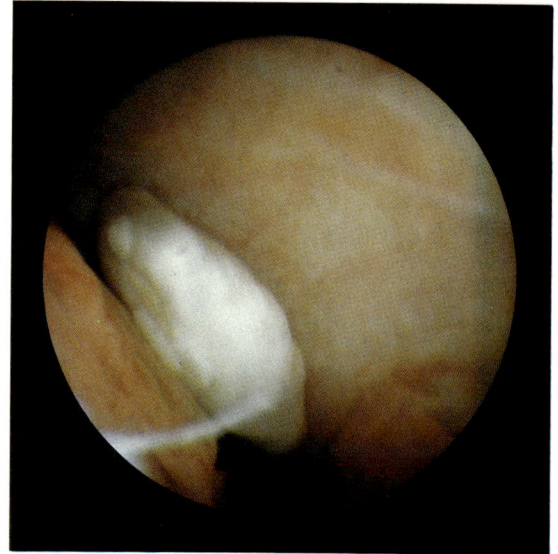

the skin. If palpation with a sterile finger in this way is unsuccessful, there is no alternative but to seek the help of the department of radiography.

Catching the loose body. When the loose body has been found it must be held still, grasped with a suitable instrument, and removed. While this is simple in theory, it is more difficult in practice because of the ease with which loose bodies can escape to the remote fastnesses of the knee.

As soon as a loose body has been sighted, the 'loose body procedure' should be put into operation. The first step is to switch off the irrigation fluid and hold the leg completely still with all escape routes blocked. The loose body will then sink to the bottom of the compartment in which it lies and come to rest. Loose bodies found in the suprapatellar pouch can be held there by an assistant's hand applied below the patella with thumb and forefinger occluding the medial and lateral gutters, which will also prevent loose bodies found in either gutter escaping into the posterior compartments (Fig. 5.4). Loose bodies in the notch will remain stationary unless disturbed by the jet of irrigation fluid from the tip of the arthroscope, the tip of the arthroscope itself or an operating instrument, and the chances of a small loose body slipping between the medial femoral condyle and the anterior cruciate ligament can be reduced still further by avoiding excessive flexion of the knee.

If the loose body lies in a gutter it can usually be pushed back up into the pouch or transfixed with a percutaneous needle, but the needle must be directed into soft tissue or articular cartilage rather than bone. Precautions against escape of the loose body should be continued while plans are made for its removal, even when it appears to be securely transfixed with a percutaneous needle (Fig. 5.5).

Removing the loose body. The technique for removing loose bodies depends on the size and number of loose bodies and on the site in which they are discovered. As a general rule, the smallest should be removed first so that the loss of saline from the knee is kept to a minimum by deferring the largest incision until last (Fig. 5.6).

1. *Small loose bodies.* Small loose bodies can be washed up the instrument cannula by placing the tip of the arthroscope against the target and withdrawing the telescope gently so that the loose body is swept along the cannula with the escaping irrigation fluid. Alternatively, the instrument can be placed against the loose body and held absolutely still while the telescope is removed and the grasping forceps passed down the cannula to seize the loose body. 'Blind' removal in this way is an unsatisfactory procedure, but can be useful in the postero-medial compartment when the loose body lies in the most dependent part of the knee and the compartment cannot be entered via the notch.

2. *Loose bodies in the suprapatellar pouch or gutters.* For larger loose bodies, the surest method of removal is to catch the loose body in the suprapatellar pouch,

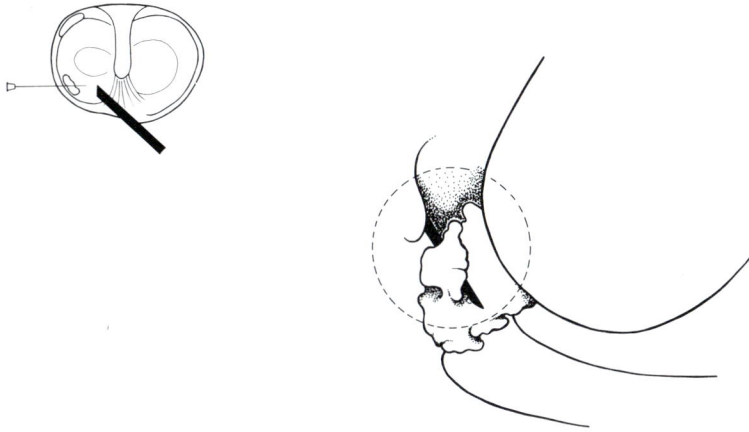

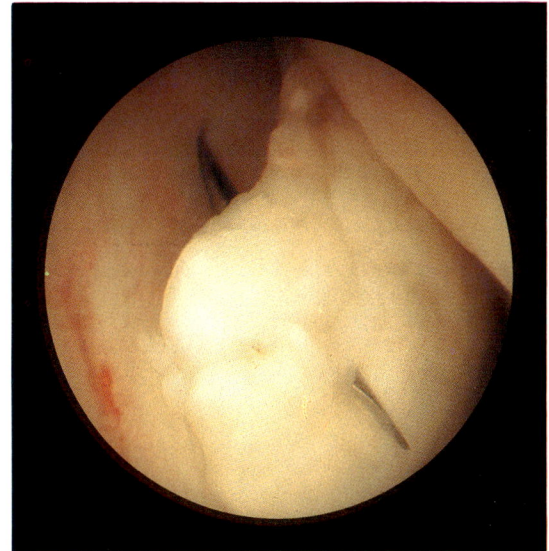

Fig. 5.5 An osteochondral fragment lying in the lateral gutter and transfixed with a percutaneous needle

lock a pair of Kocher's inserted from the lateral suprapatellar approach fairly and squarely across its middle (Fig. 5.7), and pull it out through a short skin incision. As the loose body is withdrawn, it will tent the capsule and skin which can be cut carefully with a small No. 15 blade slipped along the side of the forceps, in the manner of an episiotomy, until the knee is delivered of its burden. The forceps are easily inserted through a short incision which is conveniently made by enlarging the track created by the operating instrument cannula. It is important that the loose body is held squarely between the jaws of the forceps, because a tenuous hold on one corner will either allow it to slip away or break it into several smaller fragments.

Straight Kocher's forceps will only grasp bodies

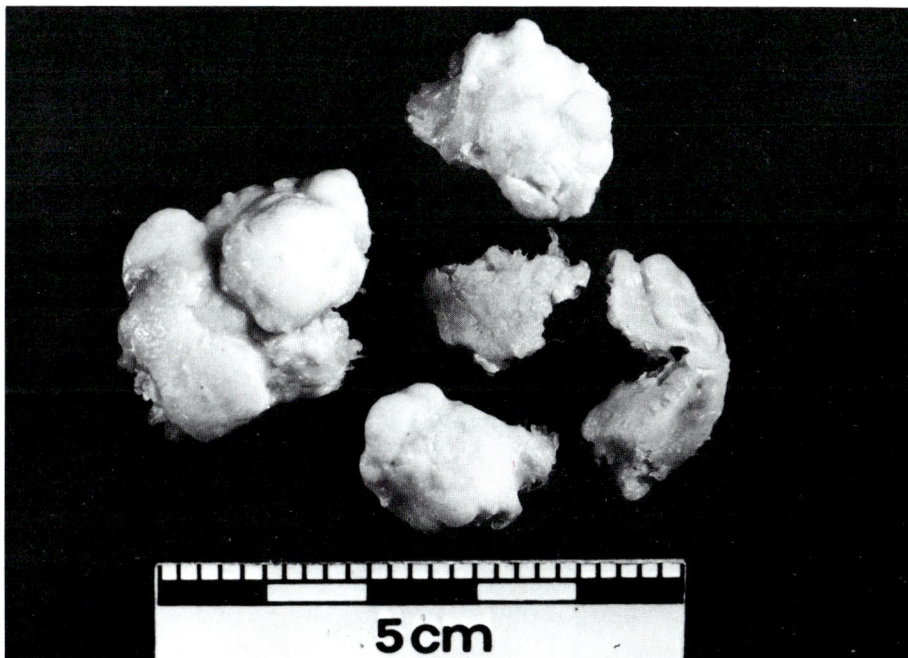

Fig. 5.6 Multiple loose bodies of differing sizes

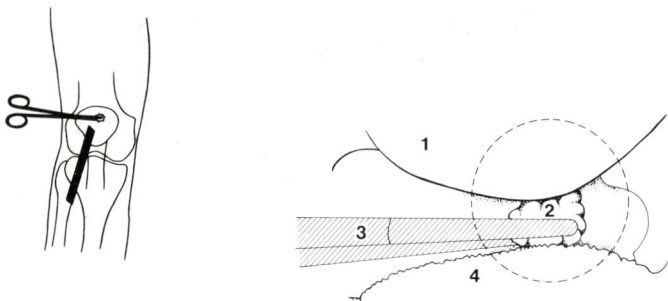

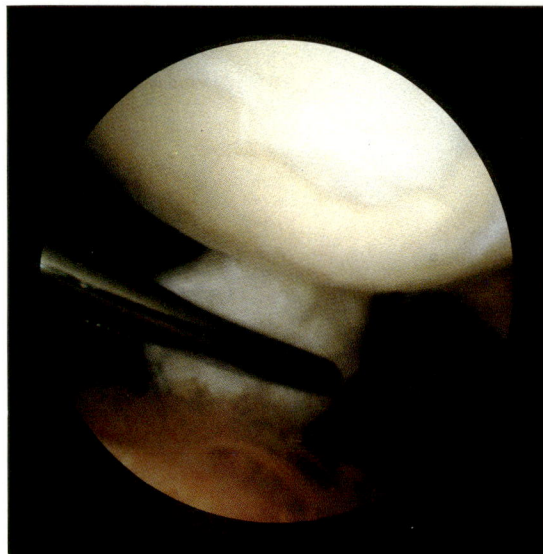

Fig. 5.7 A loose body (2) is grasped in Kocher's forceps (3) inserted from the lateral suprapatellar route; (1) patella (4) anterior surface of femur

lying in the middle of the pouch itself, and those lying in the gutters can be tantalisingly out of reach. Bouncing the loose bodies out of the gutter and into the pouch by external finger pressure will usually bring the target within the range of the forceps, but there are times when only curved instruments will be successful. Curved pituitary rongeurs are suitable provided that only gentle pressure is applied, and curved artery forceps are an alternative.

3. *Loose bodies in the intercondylar notch.* If a loose body is found in the notch, it can either be inveigled into the pouch with the arthroscope and external finger pressure or removed from the notch itself. Moving the loose body from the notch to the pouch is to run the risk of allowing it to escape into the posteromedial compartment via the medial gutter, and the decision to play the ball as it lies or attempt to move it to a better spot depends very much on the surgeon's familiarity with the postero-medial approach. If the decision is made to remove the loose body from the notch with forceps inserted from the antero-medial approach the usual problems of operating in the notch can be expected. Structures lie so close to the lens that they are difficult to assess, the fat-pad is everywhere, and the operating instruments lie uncomfortably close to the tip of the instrument. The loose body must be grasped very firmly because the capsular and subcutaneous tissues are tougher and thicker in this area than in the lateral suprapatellar

region, making it easy to lose the loose body in the subcutaneous fat. If this occurs, the loose body will not be found with the arthroscope because it lies outside the joint capsule making it necessary to open the knee. When the surgical team has re-scrubbed, re-gowned and the leg has been re-prepared and re-draped, the loose body will be found lying in the subcutaneous tissues to the delight of the nurses and the embarrassment of the surgeon.

4. *Loose bodies in the postero-medial compartment.* The average loose body will be able to elude the inexperienced surgeon and escape to the postero-medial compartment without difficulty, making an arthrotomy unavoidable unless the surgeon is experienced in manipulation of instruments inserted from the postero-medial approach. The postero-medial compartment is the most dependent part of the knee at operation so that it is very difficult for the loose body to move elsewhere, and the compartment is so small, with a well-defined inferior recess where loose bodies settle predictably, that it is actually easier to remove the loose body from the postero-medial compartment than from any other part of the knee if the surgeon is familiar with the postero-medial insertion.

If the arthroscope can be passed through the notch and the loose body identified, a percutaneous needle can be introduced and made to touch the target. The instruments are then inserted at the same point as the needle and the loose body grasped and removed either

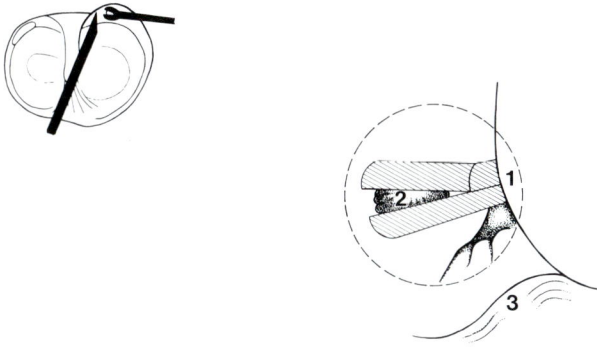

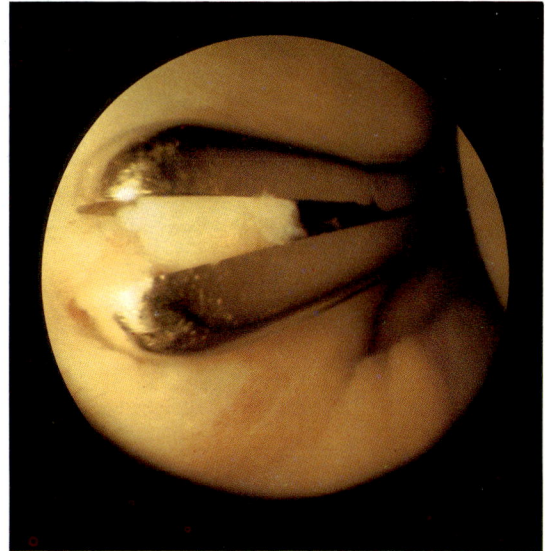

Fig. 5.8 A loose body grasped with pituitary rongeurs inserted from the postero-medial approach and seen from the antero-lateral approach (1) medial femoral condyle (2) loose body (3) medial meniscus

with Kocher's forceps or pituitary rongeurs, either straight or curved (Fig. 5.8).

If the arthroscope cannot be passed through the intercondylar notch and the loose body is found only after a postero-medial insertion of the arthroscope, it can either be removed 'blind' by passing grasping forceps down the arthroscope cannula in place of the telescope, or by passing instruments into the joint along the track of the instrument cannula and identifying the loose body by touch. The first method is successful only for small loose bodies, and the second requires such familiarity with the postero-medial approach that it is emphatically not to be attempted by beginners.

5. *Loose bodies in the postero-lateral compartment.* If the loose body comes to lie in the postero-lateral compartment or the popliteus tunnel, it can be removed with curved pituitary ronguers inserted from the lateral suprapatellar approach and passed down into the lateral gutter with the leg straight. This manoeuvre is difficult, and it may often be convenient to move the loose body to some easier area of the joint by manipulation with a hook or with a jet of saline. Large loose bodies can reach the postero-lateral compartment only through the lateral gutter, and attempts to remove them with instruments inserted through the notch or across the joint space are doomed to failure. Loose bodies that lie beneath the lateral meniscus can be removed with small angled pituitary rongeurs inserted from the antero-lateral route, with

the arthroscope transposed to the antero-medial route (Fig. 5.3).

If the leg is rested on the operating table during examination of the lateral compartment (Fig. 2.21), the postero-lateral compartment becomes the most dependent part of the knee, with the result that loose bodies gravitate towards it. The problem of loose bodies in the posterolateral compartment is not uncommon when this technique is used and it is partly to prevent foreign bodies gravitating to this region that the author prefers to examine the lateral compartment with the foot over the edge of the operating table, using the edge of the table itself as a fulcrum in the manner described in Chaper 2.

Re-examination and wound closure. When the loose body has been withdrawn, the joint should be examined again to be sure that no more loose bodies are left behind. The tourniquet can then be released, the joint irrigated and the wounds close in the usual way with one nylon suture each.

Pedunculated loose bodies

'Loose bodies' are sometimes found attached to the synovium either by fibrous adhesions (Fig. 5.9) or, in the case of osteochondral fractures, by a strip of soft tissue at the margin of the fracture. Surprisingly, these tethered loose bodies are often more difficult to remove than those which are completely loose because the pedicle or the adhesions must be divided com-

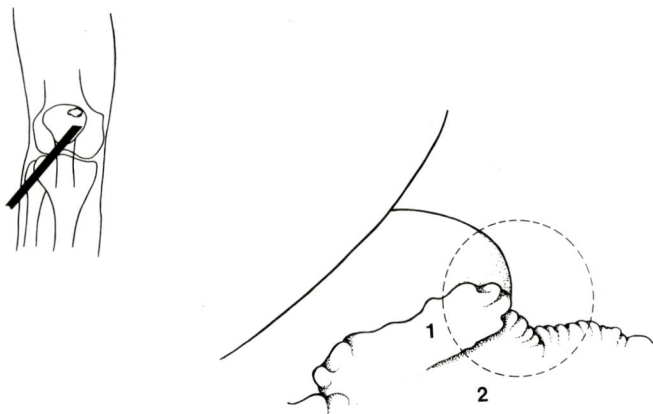

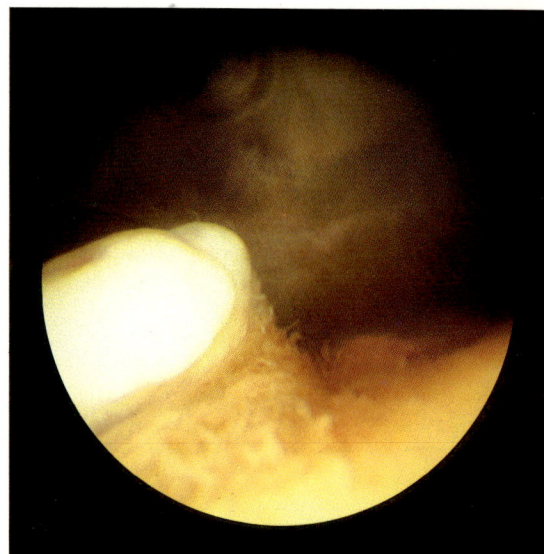

Fig. 5.9 A 'loose body' (1) which proved to be firmly adherent to the synovium (2) overlying the anterior surface of the medial femoral condyle (see Figure 5.10)

pletely before the fragment can be removed. Attempts to avulse the loose body with Kocher's forceps or rongeurs will fail because the bone of the fragment is so soft that it will itself break into fragments rather than tear the soft tissue attachment to the synovium (Fig. 5.10). If the fragment does break, the resulting crumbs of cancellous bone must be removed one by one, and any bone still adherent to the synovium picked off with pituitary rongeurs.

The stalk of a pedunculated fragment can either be

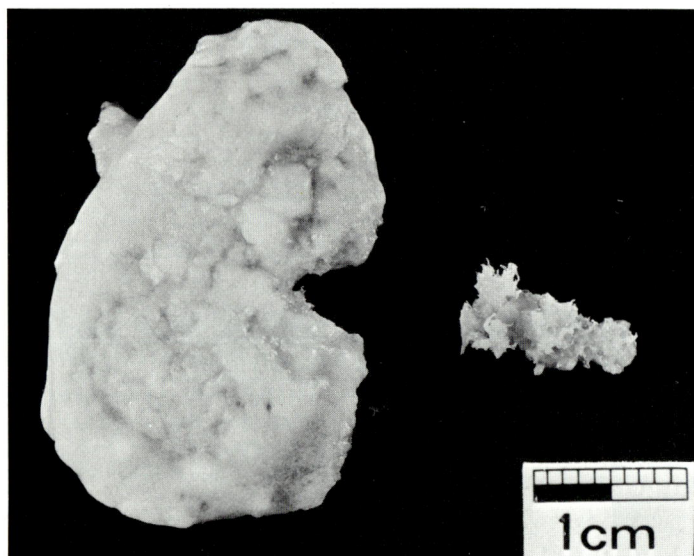

Fig. 5.10 The loose body shown in Figure 5.9, which was broken in an attempt to avulse it before it had been completely mobilised.

cut with scissors or avulsed with rongeurs, but the separation of 'loose' bodies bound down to synovium by fibrous adhesions is more difficult. Fortunately, most of these attached loose bodies lie in the suprapatellar pouch and do not need removal at all, but there are some that interfere with joint movement or cause pain. Those that do need to be removed can be mobilised with the large arthroscopic scissors and the arthroscopic knife and, when completely free in the joint, can be removed with forceps in the usual way. Because there is damage to the synovium in this procedure, the joint should be especially well irrigated before the wounds are closed.

Foreign bodies

Foreign bodies in the knee are rare, and it must be remembered that any advice offered is based on a very small experience. Most foreign bodies provoke a soft tissue reaction that tethers them to the joint wall (Fig. 5.11) with fibrous tissue which must be divided before the foreign body can be removed. If the foreign body is of a firm and smooth material such as steel or glass, the fibrous covering needs be cut at only one edge and the foreign body slipped out of its pocket, but removal of pieces of wood and fibrous material is more difficult.

Arthroscopic instruments are designed to grasp soft tissue rather than metal or glass (Fig. 5.12) and the foreign body can easily slip out of the jaws of such an instrument, usually as it is being pulled through the

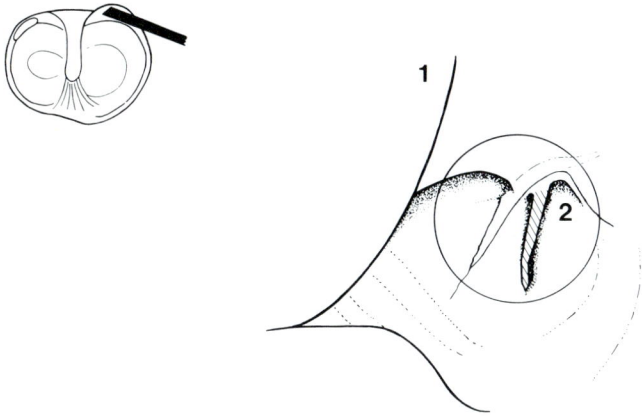

Fig. 5.11 The tip of a needle, which came to rest beneath the synovium of the posterior capsule (2), is seen from the postero-medial approach; (1) medial femoral condyle

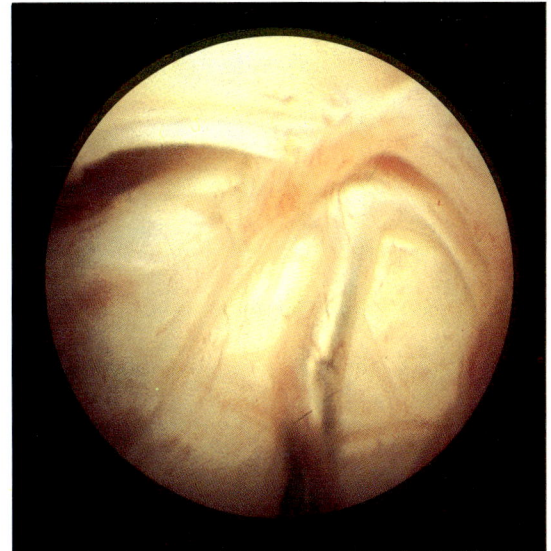

subcutaneous tissues. Apart from making a large enough hole in the subcutaneous tissue and synovium to accommodate the foreign body, and taking particular care to grasp it securely, there is no easy solution to this problem.

Chondral flaps

Isolated flaps of articular cartilage elevated from the femoral condyles or patella either extend right down to subchondral bone or involve only part of the thickness of the articular cartilage. These flaps can mimic the symptoms of a torn meniscus, and are often found unexpectedly in patients thought on clinical grounds to have a classical tear of the meniscus.

The extent of the lesion can be established with a percutaneous needle (Figs. 5.13, 5.14) and the loose fragment trimmed either through the operating arthroscope, or with rongeurs inserted through a second channel (Fig. 5.15). If the defect is large with

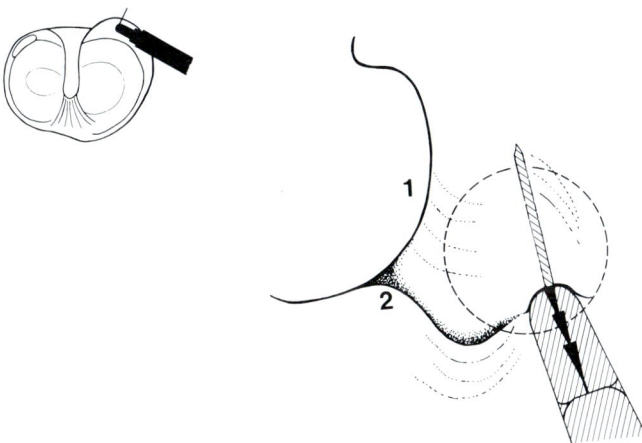

Fig. 5.12 The fragment of needle shown in Figure 5.11 is grasped in the forceps of the Wolf operating arthroscope inserted from the postero-medial approach; (1) medial femoral condyle (2) posterior edge of medial meniscus

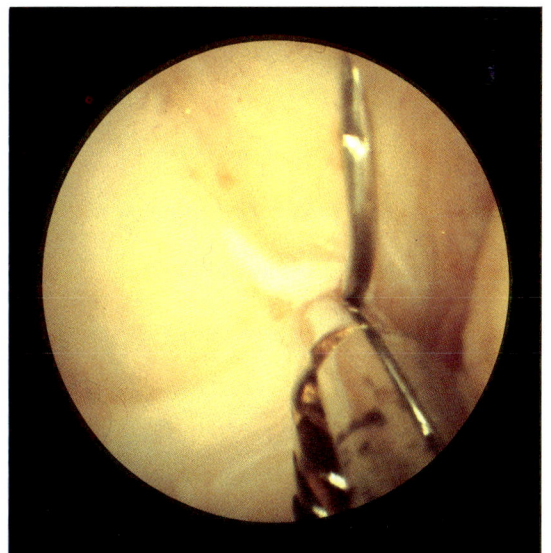

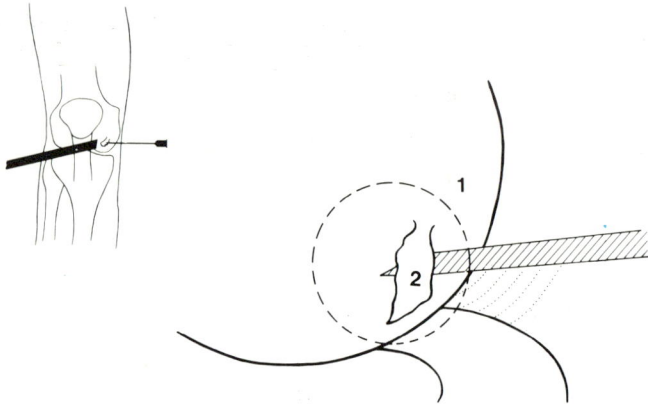

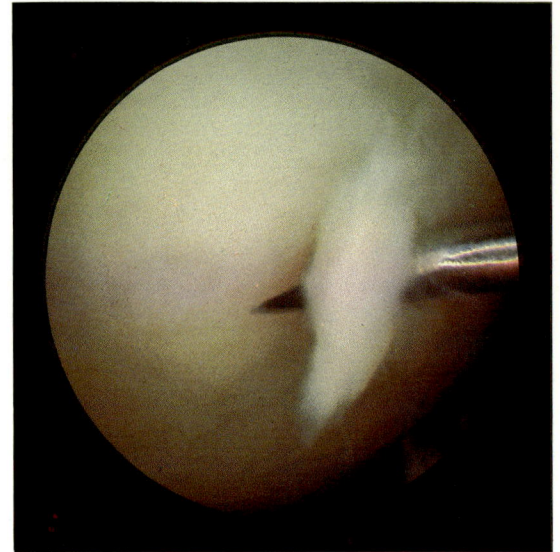

Fig. 5.13 A flap of articular cartilage (2) raised from the medial femoral condyle (1) is manipulated with a percutaneous needle inserted from the antero-medial approach

exposed subchondral bone, the problem is considerable and there is little chance of preventing the eventual onset of osteoarthritis. One solution is to drill through the base of these craters into cancellous bone with a power operated drill passed along the instrument cannula, or with a Kirschner wire passed directly through the skin (Fig. 5.16). The flow of irrigation fluid washes most of the debris down the cannula alongside the drill and out of the knee and any residual debris must be removed by thorough irrigation. The

post-operative care does not differ from that required for an open drilling of bone except that the patient can leave hospital within 24 hours of operation.

Subchondral bone necrosis

There is no satisfactory treatment for subchondral bone necrosis, in which the bony defect is covered only by a layer of articular cartilage that can be popped in and out on the end of the telescope like a dent on a

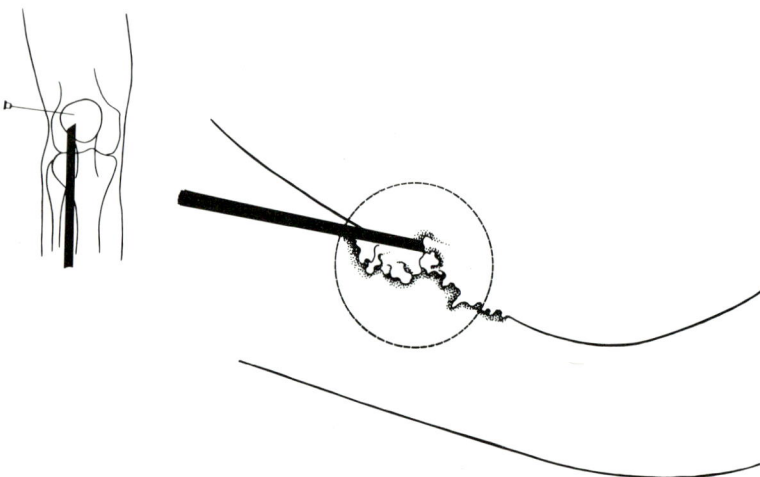

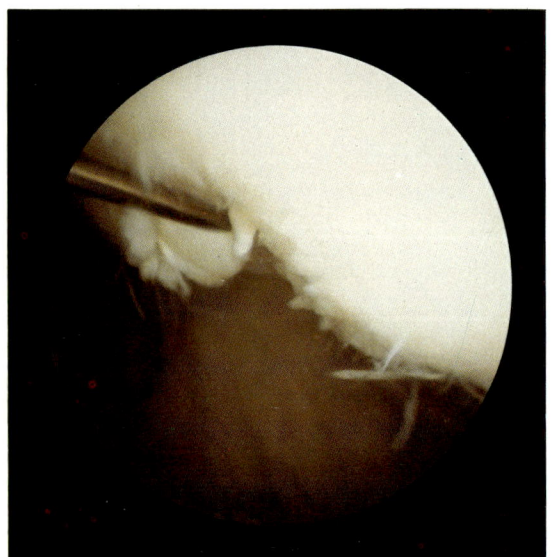

Fig. 5.14 Probing a chondral fracture of the lateral margin of the patella using the irrigation needle

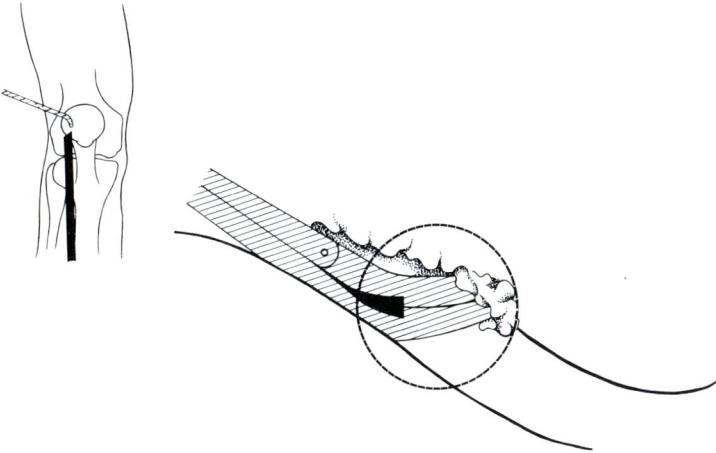

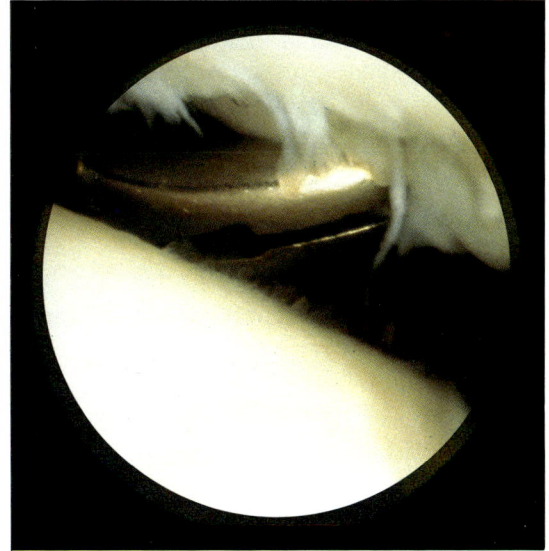

Fig. 5.15 Trimming the chondral fracture shown in Figure 5.14 using curved pituitary rongeurs

ping-pong ball. These lesions are common in patients who have received renal transplants, and in others who have received large doses of steroids. Although unroofing the bony defect by excising the cartilage covering and then drilling its base is a simple and elegant arthroscopic procedure, there is no evidence that it does any good to the patient, and these lesions are perhaps best left well alone.

Osteochondritis dissecans

As the name implies, osteochondritis dissecans is a chronic process and must be distinguished from an acute osteochondral fracture. The gradual dissection and separation of a fragment of bone from the medial wall of the intercondylar notch is associated with pain and discomfort most marked when the knee is

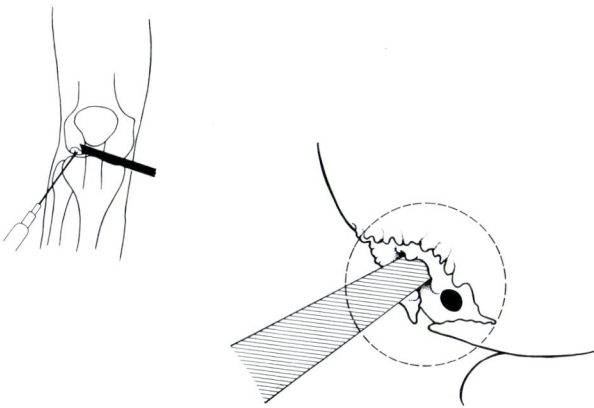

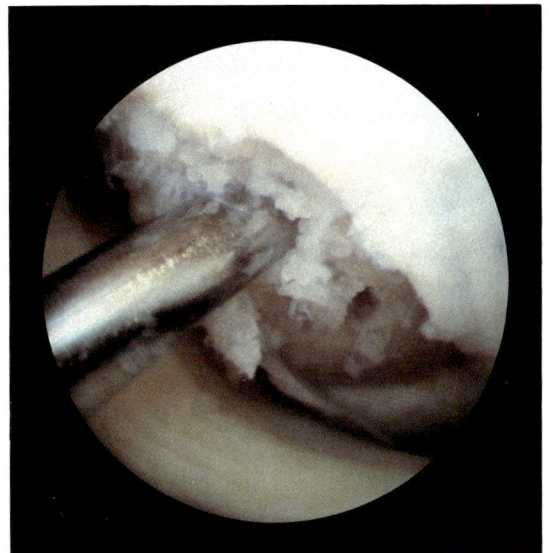

Fig. 5.16 Drilling the subchondral bed of a full thickness chondral fracture of the lateral femoral condyle with a thick Kirschner wire

extended and the tibia rotated internally. Early lesions can be identified arthroscopically by a linear defect in the articular cartilage, marking the edge of the loose fragment. As the pathological process advances the block of bone is extruded gradually from the femur and comes to stand proud of the surrounding cartilage where it can be manipulated with a percutaneous needle. Later still, the fragment will separate as a loose body when the surface of both the loose body and crater quickly acquire a cartilaginous covering that makes it impossible to replace the fragment precisely.

Although the early bone changes of dissecans lesions can be seen easily on the radiographs, the early articular cartilage changes can be difficult to find at athroscopy. Gentle probing with a hook or needle will usually detect areas of softening and dimming the light source by turning down the voltage with the control knob, or more simply by loosening the attachments of the light cable to the arthroscope, will often show up irregularities in the joint surface that were not previously apparent. The injection of methylene blue into the joint has also been advocated as an aid to the recognition of softened articular cartilage, but few surgeons have found it helpful.

The ideal time for treating an area of osteochondritis is before the bone has separated completely, when it can be reattached with Kirschner wires drilled through the fragment into the underlying femur from the antero-lateral approach. The wires can then be advanced until they protrude through the skin on the medial side of the knee, and withdrawn further under arthroscopic control until their tips lie just beneath the articular cartilage. The knee should then be immobilised in plaster for 6–8 weeks while the fragment becomes reattached, the wires removed, and physiotherapy instituted.

Sadly, patients with fragments suitable for re-attachment in this way are less common than those who present when the fragment has separated completely from its underlying bed. While it is perfectly possible to screw such fragments back into their bed and even to insert bone grafts under arthroscopic control, such procedures must be followed by a period of plaster immobilisation of several weeks. The great advantage of arthroscopic surgery is early mobilisation and in the author's opinion there is no point in performing a procedure arthroscopically unless it enables the knee to be mobilised more quickly or makes it possible for the procedure to be completed more precisely and effectively than by other means.

Neither of these conditions apply to the screwing and grafting of osteochondritis dissecans lesions.

Osteochondral fractures

Acute osteochondral fractures should be diagnosed clinically and with the help of radiographs, but arthroscopy is helpful to clear the haemarthrosis and inspect the joint. It is possible to replace the fragment of an acute osteochondral fragment in its bed accurately and secure it with pins or screws arthroscopically, but the operation is simpler if the joint is open. On one occasion when the joint was opened to reattach an osteochondral fragment that had arisen from the lateral edge of the lateral femoral condyle, the fragment was found to include only a very thin layer of bone which proved too flimsy for any kind of accurate fixation. Attempts at fixation were abandoned and the fragment discarded. Removal of the fragment arthroscopically would have allowed it to be examined and its suitability for reattachment to be assessed without opening the joint needlessly and on the basis of this experience, removal of the fragment arthroscopically is recommended so that it can be examined carefully before the knee is opened.

The screws and pins used for internal fixation of osteochondral fragments can also be removed arthroscopically. Screws are removed more easily than Smillie's pins, which become deeply buried and cannot be grasped easily with the arthroscopic instruments. When removing screws, time should be spent determining the best point of insertion of the instruments by flexing the knee until the screw head can be reached easily from either the antero-lateral or antero-medial approach with a percutaneous needle, and a short incision then made at that point to admit the screwdriver.

Trimming, shaving and drilling

Irregularities of the articular cartilage of the patella or femoral condyle can be levelled with rongeurs, basket forceps or a powered shaver. The indications for articular cartilage shaving are controversial, but have extended noticeably since it became possible to perform the procedure arthroscopically.

In general, it appears that the 'crab meat' lesions with a localised area of flaking articular cartilage fare better after shaving than the finer fibrillation or generalised irregularity associated with degenerative joint disease. The lesions suitable for shaving are comparatively rare and the author is in no doubt that many patellae are being shaved quite unnecessarily for no better reason than that the surgeon is the proud possessor of a powered shaver.

Anything that can be done to localised articular cartilage lesions at arthrotomy can also be done arthroscopically so that it is now possible to analyse the effects of the intra-articular procedure without the additional trauma of arthrotomy. The results of such studies can be expected to throw much-needed light on the management of these lesions.

Trimming with rongeurs and basket forceps

Pituitary rongeurs or basket forceps can be used to level areas of irregularity and upcutting rongeurs can be used to remove all softened articular cartilage until subchondral bone is exposed and the edges of the lesion are vertical, which is not possible with the powered shaver. If desired, holes can be drilled down to the underlying cancellous bone through the subchondral bed.

A knife can also be used to level the cartilage, but the use of a knife makes it impossible to avoid damage to healthy articular cartilage at the margin of the lesion and the use of the knife in this procedure is not recommended.

Powered shavers

The shaver inserted through a trocar and cannula from the suprapatellar approach can be brought to bear on the patella or femoral condyle by manipulation of the instrument, the patella, and the femur. It is sensible to touch the target area with the tip of the irrigation needle before inserting the shaver to make certain that the target area can be reached from the intended point of insertion.

The shaver must be attached to a suction apparatus and the vacuum adjusted until a gentle stream of saline is drawn slowly into the instrument. If the suction is too strong the rate of outflow will exceed the rate of inflow, the synovial cavity will deflate, and the examination will become impossible. This difficulty can be overcome by reducing the vacuum, increasing the rate of inflow by elevation of the reservoir or irrigation fluid, or injecting the irrigation fluid under pressure. A simple filter in the form of a gauze swab placed over the end of the outflow tube where it enters

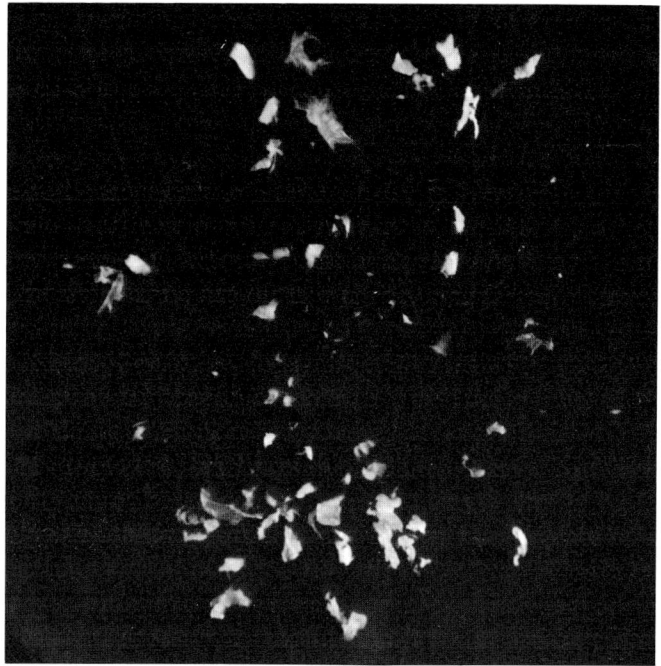

Fig. 5.17 Articular cartilage shavings obtained with the Dyonics shaver

the suction bottle will retain the harvest of cartilage fragments for later inspection (Fig. 5.17).

The shaver is so designed that its side-cutting window will only remove tissue that stands proud of its surroundings, but it is still possible to remove the superficial layers of healthy articular cartilage through clumsy handling and it is essential with this instrument, as with all others, to keep the cutting tip in view at all times (Fig. 5.18). To use the instrument 'blind' is very likely to cause grievous damage to structures that would be better preserved intact.

Some surgeons point out that shaving the patella is not a particularly effective operation when done through an arthrotomy and that there is no reason to suppose the results will be any better if the procedure is done arthroscopically, but in favour of arthroscopic shaving it must be said that it adds little to the trauma of arthroscopy. When the surgeon has become good at arthroscopic surgery, there is a temptation to think that any arthroscopic operation must be good and, as Dr R W Jackson has commented, when you only have a hammer, most things look like nails. Only time will tell if the long-term results of arthroscopic shaving justify the procedure.

Drilling

Articular cartilage lesions of the patella and femur,

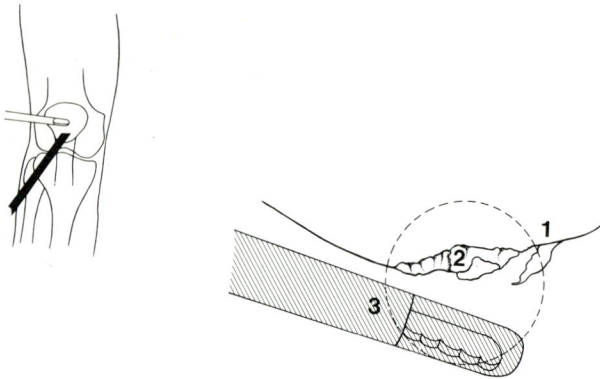

Fig. 5.18 An irregularity (2) on the under-surface of the patella (1) after levelling with the patellar shaver (3)

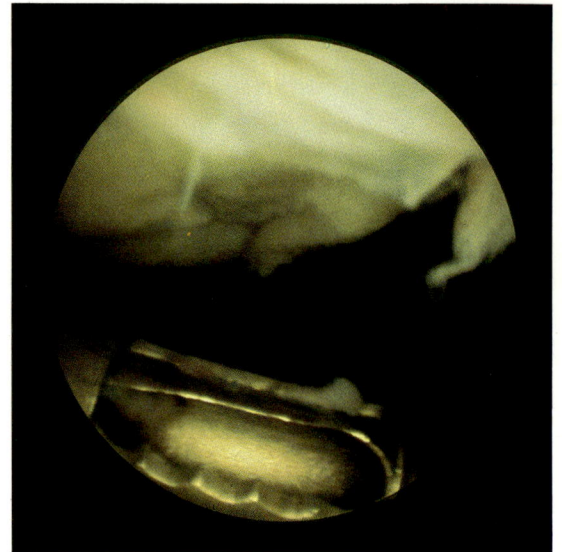

like chondral flaps, can also be treated by drilling through the articular cartilage and subchondral bone into cancellous bone using a drill bit passed along the instrument cannula, or a Kirschner wire inserted directly through the skin (Fig. 5.16). The drill holes can be made into cancellous bone either directly through the damaged articular cartilage itself (Fig. 5.19) or into the subchondral bone after removal of the overlying cartilage with pituitary rongeurs.

To pass a long Kirschner wire down the instrument channel of the operating arthroscope is also possible,

but this technique makes the procedure needlessly difficult and imposes serious restrictions on the angle at which the hole can be drilled.

The 'impingement' lesion

The articular cartilage defect found at the point of impingement of the medial femoral condyle and the anterior horn of the meniscus has already been mentioned (Fig. 2.18, 2.19). This lesion, which is often associated with a painful hyperextension jerk

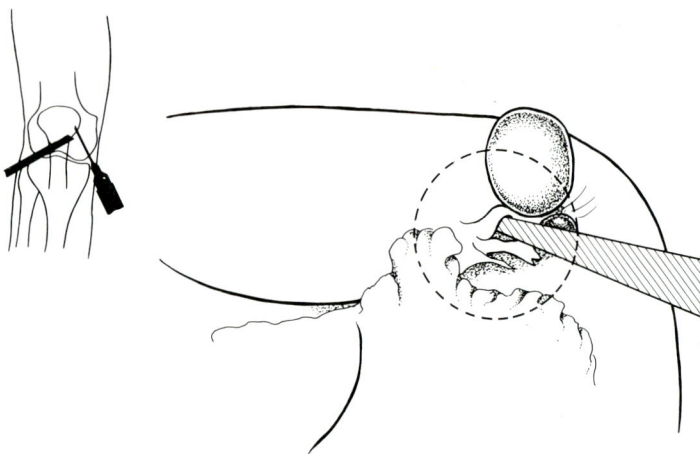

Fig. 5.19 Drilling into cancellous bone through a patch of softened and degenerate articular cartilage on the medial facet of the patella using a percutaneous Kirschner wire

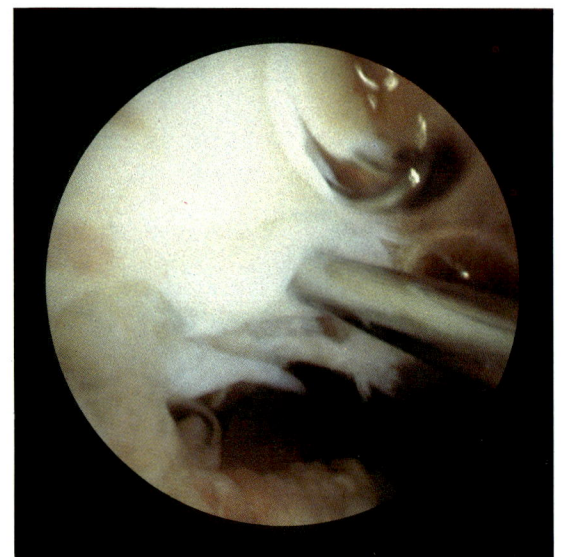

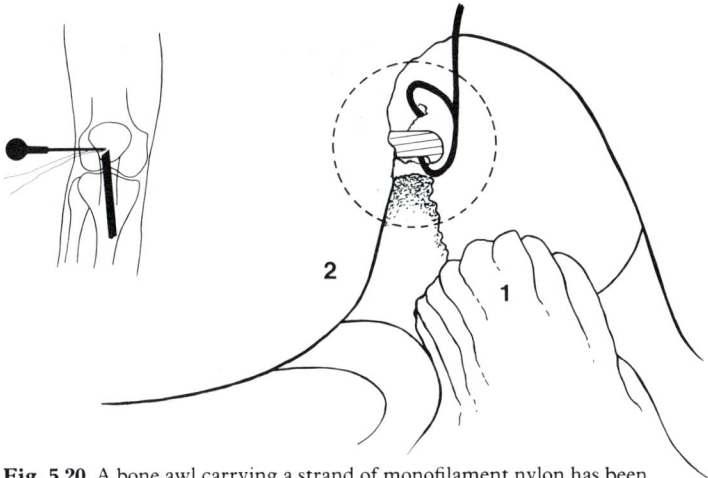

Fig. 5.20 A bone awl carrying a strand of monofilament nylon has been passed through the lateral femoral condyle to the site of attachment of a ruptured anterior cruciate ligament (1). The nylon can then be used to draw a carbon fibre replacement for the anterior cruciate ligament through the lateral condyle (2)

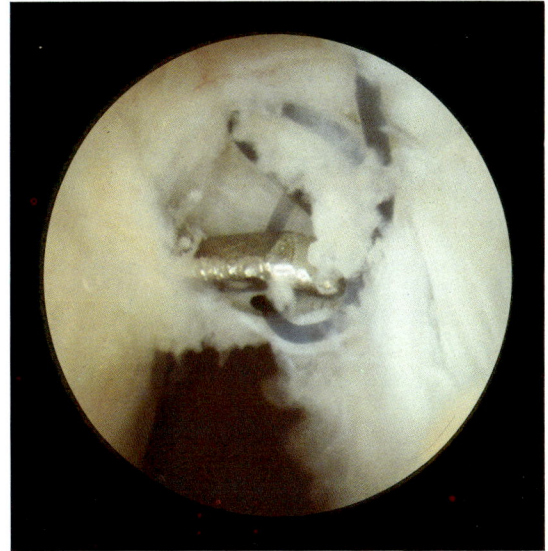

and the synovial fold syndrome, is also found in young atheletes who exercise to excess. The lesion can be trimmed with the basket forceps of the operating arthroscope as an adjunct to the division of the synovial shelf, but a ragged base will be left and it is very probable that the lesion will reform unless the patient modifies his training regime. The full significance of this lesion is not yet known.

Ligament lesions

The arthroscope makes possible a dynamic assessment of meniscal movement when the anterior or posterior drawer sign is positive, and is also helpful in the assessment of lax ligaments (Fig. 2.33) and lesions in continuity.

Although at present the main use of the arthroscope in the management of ligament lesions lies in diagnosis and assessment, its role in the future is likely to be more important. To insert a replacement cruciate ligament of a material such as carbon fibre under arthroscopic control and without the need for arthrotomy is now a simple matter (Figs. 5.20, 5.21) and the

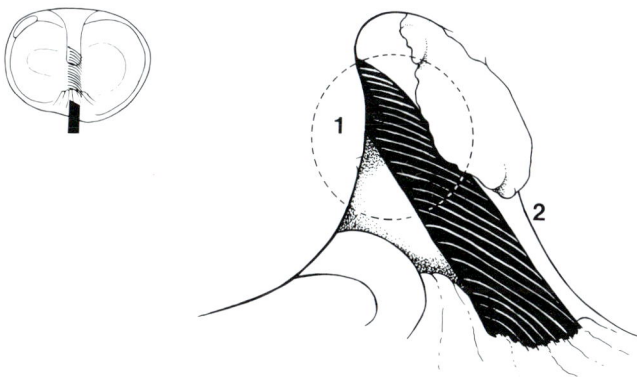

Fig. 5.21 A carbon fibre replacement of the anterior cruciate ligament lying in the intercondylar notch. The carbon fibre was inserted under arthroscopic control. (1) Lateral femoral condyle (2) medial femoral condyle

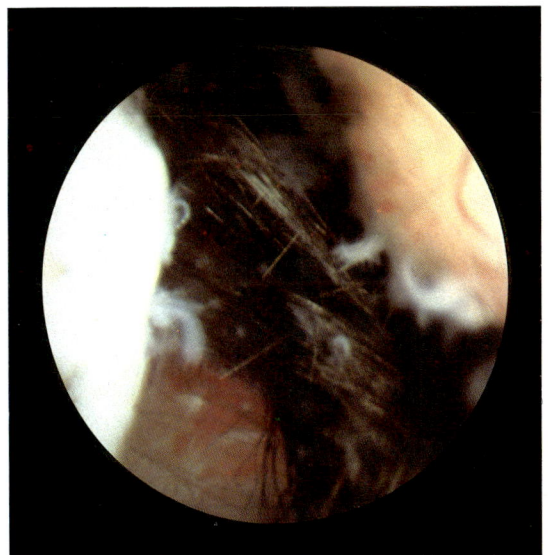

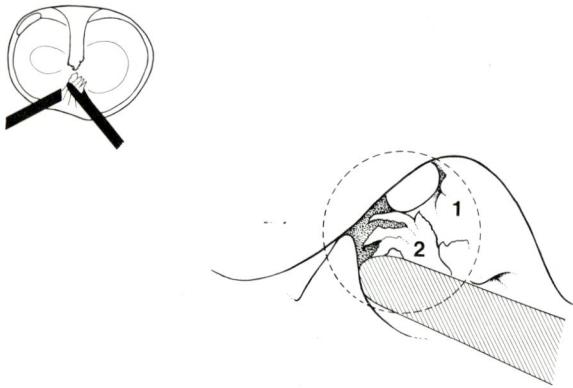

Fig. 5.22 The redundant stub of a ruptured anterior cruciate ligament (2) is removed from the intercondylar notch (1) using pituitary rongeurs inserted from the antero-medial route

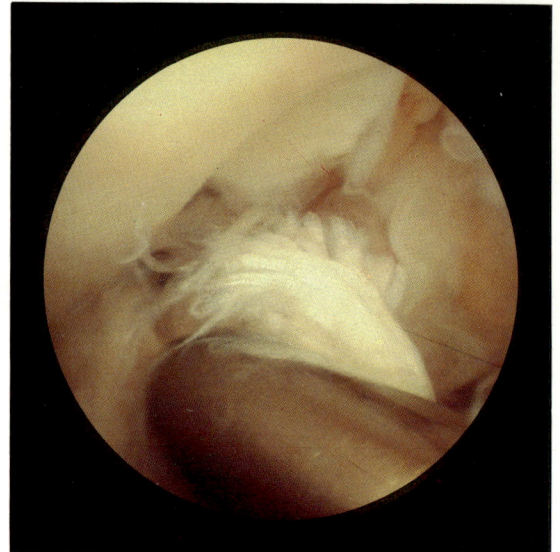

presence of an intact capsule makes it possible to adjust the tension of the material more precisely than was previously possible. At present the knee must still be immobilised in plaster for some weeks after replacement of the cruciate ligament, and an extra-capsular repair is usually advisable as an additional procedure, but the time when a patient's knee can be restrung with a new cruciate ligament as an out-patient procedure may not be too far distant. The surgical technique is already available, and awaits the development of the appropriate material.

Anterior cruciate stubs

If the anterior cruciate ruptures at its proximal femoral attachment, a long stub of tissue will remain. These stubs may be over 2 cm in length, are quite long enough to cause mechanical symptoms and sometimes become so thickened and oedematous that they cause a painful block to extension.

The stub, which is functionally useless, is easily removed with instruments inserted from the antero-medial approach and can be trimmed back to its base

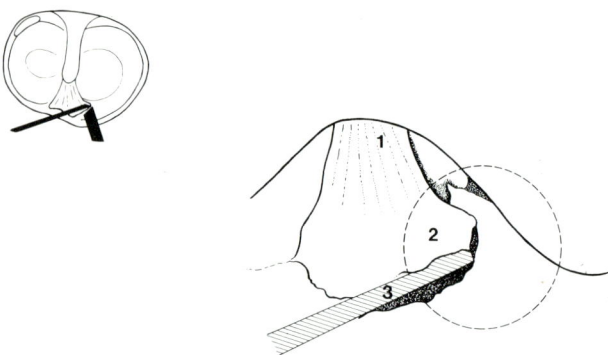

Fig. 5.23 Avulsion of tibial spine. The anterior cruciate ligament (1) has avulsed a block of bone including the tibial spine (2) from the underlying tibia, and is manipulated with a probing hook (3) inserted from the antero-lateral route with the arthroscope inserted from the antero-medial route

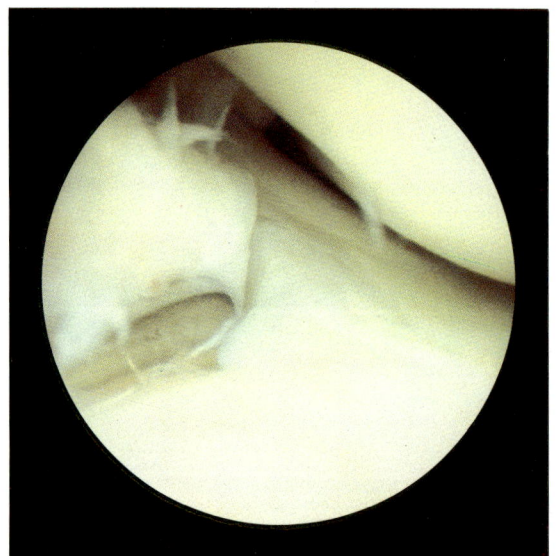

with ease using punch forceps or rongeurs (Fig. 5.22). The procedure is simple and well within the grasp of a cautious beginner.

Avulsed tibial fragments

If the anterior cruciate ligament avulses a fragment of bone from the tibia, the fragment can come to lie in the intercondylar notch and block full extension of the knee. If this fracture is diagnosed early the fragment can be reattached either surgically or by plaster immobilisation but if found later, either the bed of the fracture can be deepened and the fragment reattached—a difficult procedure with a dubious outcome—or the fragment can be excised arthroscopically. Arthroscopic excision is not difficult, but like other operations in the intercondylar notch, the instruments and target lie close to the lens and create the usual difficulties. The fragment should first be mobilised with a long-handled knife and small periosteal elevator so that it can be removed with curved and straight pituitary rongeurs (Fig. 5.23). The operation is easier if the arthroscope is transferred to the antero-medial approach and the instruments inserted from the antero-lateral route.

6

Operations on meniscal lesions

A. INTRODUCTION

The purpose of this chapter is to describe how damaged menisci can be treated without arthrotomy, but a brief outline of the role of arthroscopy in the assessment and management of meniscal lesions is necessary as an introduction.

Assessment

As already mentioned in Chapter 2, the clinical history is more important in the assessment of any knee disorder than clinical examination, plain radiography, arthrography, and arthroscopy combined. The patient's account of his symptoms and their onset will usually enable the clinician to decide if the underlying pathology involves synovium, ligaments, articular cartilage or meniscus, and in which compartment of the knee the pathology is present.

The arthroscopist will quickly find that geniune meniscal lesions are less common than he had been led to believe. The symptoms associated with a true meniscus lesion can usually be attributed to the mechanical effects of the loose meniscal fragment when the knee is flexed and twisted without great external violence, often during such gentle activities as putting on a pair of shoes or rising from the kneeling position. These symptoms can readily be distinguished from sudden episodes of instability when the patient applies great stress to the knee, such as occur when twisting sharply during a game of football and which are usually associated with ligament injuries. The predominantly mechanical nature of the problems that follow a meniscal injury is hardly surprising when it is remembered that because the

body of the meniscus has no sensory nerve supply it cannot itself be the seat of pain or tenderness, and in this respect a loose meniscal fragment can readily be compared with a loose body, from which it differs only by being tethered at the jointline. Although a distorted meniscus can stretch synovium or capsule and give rise to pain and tenderness at the jointline, these features seldom overshadow the repeated episodes of locking or jamming that are the essential features of a true meniscal lesion.

The importance of the meniscus

There is an increasing body of evidence to support the concept that the meniscus is an essential part of the mechanical structure of the knee. Oretorp (1978) has shown that the peripheral fibres of the medial meniscus blend intimately with the medial ligament, and that to perform a total medial meniscectomy is to excise part of the medial collateral ligament complex. Seedhom, Dowson and Wright (1974) have reported that the medial meniscus transmits 50 per cent and the lateral meniscus 75 per cent of the load across the joint when the knee is straight.

Histological study of the menisci shows that they are essentially complex ligaments (Bullough et al 1970) differing from other ligaments in their fine structure, ground substance and in the smooth surface that is necessary because the meniscus must articulate with the surface of the femur and tibia. The crescentic shape of the menisci also sets them apart from other ligaments, but is essential for meniscal function because the firm attachment to bone at each end allows the circumferentially disposed fibres to act as a hoop, resisting the bursting force imposed by the downward thrust of the femoral condyle. By removing this protective shock-absorbing hoop, particularly in the lateral compartment, total meniscectomy increases the load taken by the articular cartilage and can only accelerate degenerative joint changes.

The importance of degenerative joint disease following meniscectomy is more than a theoretical consideration. As Huckell (1965) has pointed out, meniscectomy is not a benign procedure, and 30 per cent of patients may show some clinical symptoms and signs of degenerative arthritis within 10 years of operation. Similar findings have been reported by Gear (1967), and J P Jackson (1968). The protagonists of wholesale routine meniscectomy say that it is impossible to distinguish between the long-term ill-effects of the injury that led to the meniscal lesion, the effect of a loose meniscal fragment in the knee, the trauma of operation, and the absence of the meniscus itself. These criticisms cannot be levelled at the work of Zaman and Leonard (1978), who have shown that the long-term effects of removing normal menisci from children are poor, with over 70 per cent developing the clinical and radiological features of osteoarthritis in the second or third decades of life.

With this and other evidence available, there is no longer any reason to regard the meniscus as an unnecessary and troublesome appendage that can be excised with impunity, and it might even be argued that excision of a normal meniscus is a surgical error comparable with the amputation of a normal finger.

Selective surgery of the meniscus

Meniscal lesions can be treated by reattachment of the meniscal fragment, excision of the fragment or complete excision of the whole meniscus, and all of these procedures have enjoyed periods of popularity in the past which have come and gone with the tides of surgical fashion. Many lesions, such as minor splits or fissures that cannot be related to the patient's symptoms, can be left well alone and the belief that any one operation is the correct solution for all meniscal lesions is a dangerous over-simplification that should be replaced by careful selection of the appropriate operation for each type of lesion.

Reattachment of the meniscal fragment with catgut was first described by Annandale in 1885, but the recurrence of symptoms was so frequent that the procedure was soon replaced by excision of the loose fragment (Jones R 1909). Reattachment of the meniscus is now being re-examined (Stone R 1979) and may well be the treatment of choice for separations of the anterior horn and peripheral tears of the medial meniscus that involve the vascular rim of tissue at the menisco-synovial junction. At present, meniscal re-attachment ('meniscoresis') is usually followed by plaster immobilisation so that there is no great advantage in reattaching the meniscus arthroscopically.

Excision of localised 'bucket handle' fragments of meniscus has never fallen entirely from favour, despite the protestations of some that the symptoms recur unless the intact rim is also excised. While excision of the bucket handle is recognised as an acceptable procedure, there has been less enthusiasm for the open excision of isolated flaps or tags of meniscus, but it is hard to find a sensible reason for excision of the remaining healthy meniscus if the symptoms are due only to an isolated flap or tag. The aim of partial meniscectomy, performed by either open or arthroscopic techniques, is to leave an intact and stable rim of healthy tissue. Multiple tears of the meniscus are common, and to remove one bucket handle while leaving another is to perform an incomplete rather than a partial meniscectomy. Great care must always be taken to ensure that the remaining meniscal tissue is intact and stable.

We are at present emerging from a period when total meniscectomy enjoyed widespread popularity and there are now several reports comparing the early and late results of partial and total meniscectomy (Bonnin 1956, Tapper and Hoover 1969, McGinty, Geuss and Marvin 1977), all favouring partial meniscectomy. Not only is partial meniscectomy a simpler operation than total meniscectomy whether performed arthroscopically or at arthrotomy, but the post-operative rehabilitation is shorter and the long-term results are better. These reports are encouraging to arthroscopists who have become increasingly sceptical of the clinical importance of some of the meniscal lesions for which total meniscectomy has been performed. Tiny fissures and irregularities in the meniscus are by no means uncommon and often seen in patients whose symptoms arise from obvious disorders elsewhere in the knee, and degenerative changes in the meniscus are almost universal in patients with early degenerative osteoarthritis in whom, despite the presence of a few splits or fissures, the meniscus may well be the healthiest structure in the knee. It is difficult to understand how excision of such a meniscus can do anything but accelerate the degenerate process by increasing the load upon the already damaged articular surface, and such menisci should probably be left undisturbed (Jones, Smith and Reisch 1978).

The suggestion has sometimes been made (Smillie, 1970) that total excision of the meniscal rim leads to regeneration of a new meniscus. Although a small whitish crescent will develop at the site of the former meniscus histological study of this structure shows that it consists only of flimsy fibrous tissue and bears nothing more than a superficial macroscopic resemblance to the original meniscus. In contrast, Hargreaves and Seedhom (1979) have shown that the intact rim left after removing a bucket handle fragment is capable of transmitting 35 per cent of the load across the joint.

Although total meniscectomy is deservedly in decline as a routine procedure for all meniscal tears, it is still the treatment of choice for cystic degeneration of the meniscus. Although isolated peripheral cysts of the lateral meniscus can easily be excised without disturbing the peripheral fibres of the meniscus, the whole of the meniscus must be removed when it is degenerate and swollen throughout its substance. Total or subtotal meniscectomy is also required if the meniscal rim is completely ruptured or if the meniscus is so badly torn that no healthy meniscal tissue can be identified.

Classification of meniscal lesions

The selective approach to meniscal surgery demands that the exact anatomy of the lesion is identified before the appropriate operation is selected. If the decision is made to perform a partial or subtotal meniscectomy arthroscopically, the operation should proceed in three stages:

1. Identification of the exact anatomy of the lesion;
2. Removal of the fragment;
3. Trimming the rim and checking its stability.

Of these three stages, the identification of the exact anatomy is the most important, the removal of the meniscal fragment the easiest, and checking the rim the most difficult. Because the anatomy of the lesion is so important, the preliminary arthroscopy will usually need to include the use of a percutaneous needle, a probing hook, or a second insertion of the arthroscope. The information obtained from a com-

plete arthroscopy should be sufficient to place the meniscus lesion in one of several categories so that the appropriate method of excision can be selected.

Experience of arthroscopic surgery is still limited and the classification offered is a prototype that will inevitably be expanded and improved. It is not put forward as a definitive catalogue of meniscal pathology, but has nevertheless proved quite satisfactory in practice.

B. MEDIAL MENISCUS

Tears of the medial meniscus can be broadly divided into circumferential tears which give rise to bucket handle fragments, flaps and tags arising from horizontal tears, degenerative lesions found in patients with osteoarthrosis, and a variety of miscellaneous lesions. The identification of one lesion does not exclude the presence of others and the existence of double, triple and even quadruple tears must always be remembered, as must the possibility of the patient having more than one type of tear in either or both menisci.

Circumferential tears

Circumferential tears of the medial meniscus originate in the posterior horn, either at the posterior insertion of the meniscus or very close to it, and extend anteriorly for a variable distance to produce a bucket handle fragment. For practical purposes, bucket handle fragments of the medial meniscus always extend right up to the posterior insertion, however far anteriorly they may run, and can be divided conveniently into three types, according to the extent of the tear.

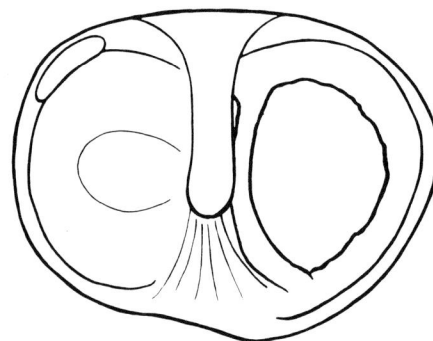

Fig. 6.1 Complete (Type 1) bucket handle tear of the medial meniscus, with the tear extending right up to the anterior attachment and the fragment lying in the intercondylar notch

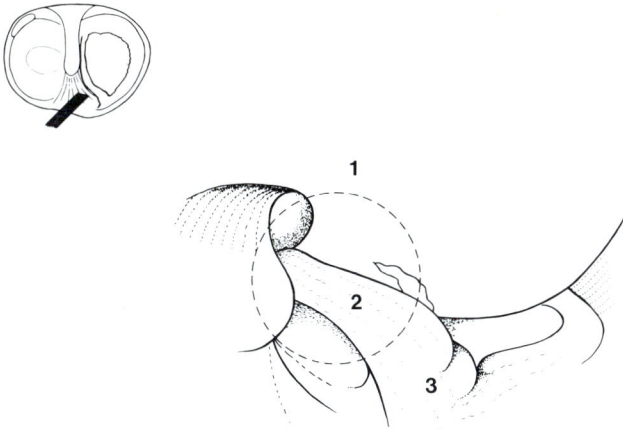

Fig. 6.2 A complete (Type 1) bucket handle tear of the medial meniscus (2) lying locked in the intercondylar notch beneath the medial femoral condyle (1). The anterior attachment of the fragment (3) is at the anterior horn of the medial meniscus

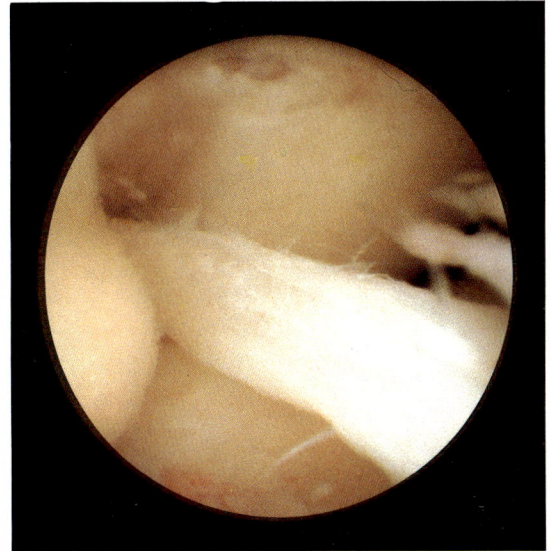

Complete (Type 1) circumferential tears. If the circumferential split extends right up to the anterior insertion, the bucket handle fragment will come to lie easily in the intercondylar notch (Figs. 6.1, 6.2). Tears of this pattern may cause remarkably few symptoms and the fragment can sometimes lie so comfortably in the intercondylar notch that a full range of extension is still possible. Even when some loss of extension is present, the knee may gradually straighten over a period of years as the surrounding

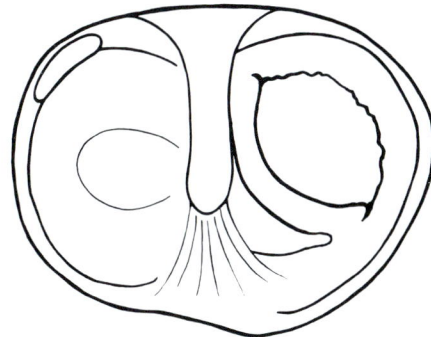

Fig. 6.3 Incomplete (Type 2) bucket handle tear of the medial meniscus, with the anterior limit of the tear falling short of the anterior attachment

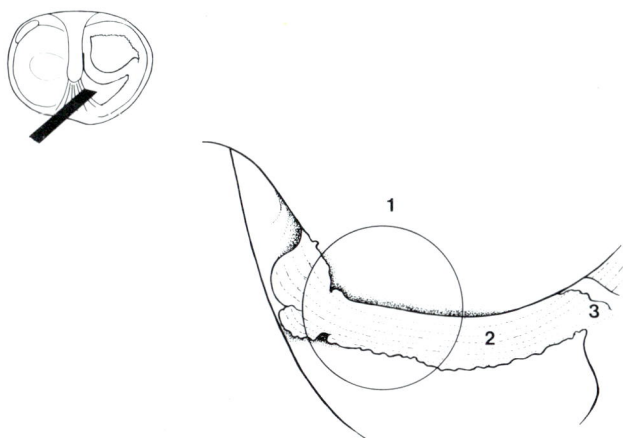

Fig. 6.4 An incomplete (Type 2) bucket handle tear of the medial meniscus (2) with the anterior limit of the tear (3) falling short of the anterior attachment—(1) medial femoral condyle

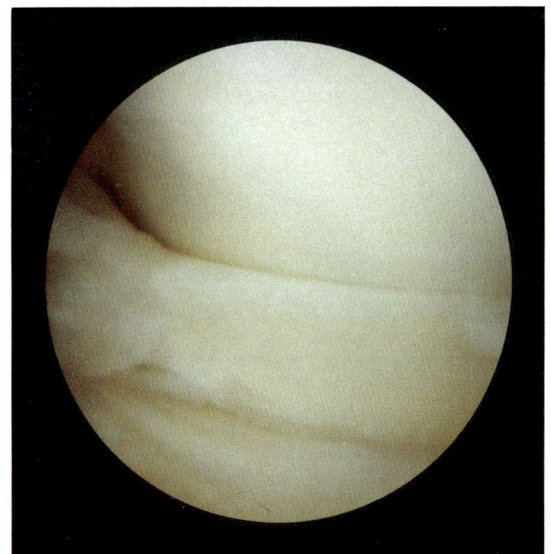

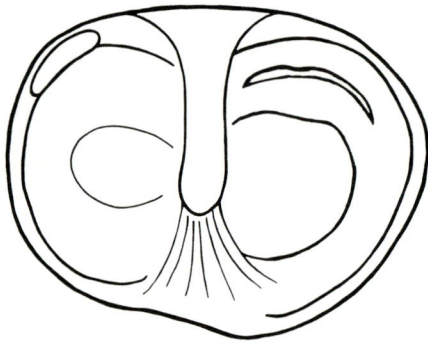

Fig. 6.5 Concealed (Type 3) circumferential tear of the medial meniscus lying in the posterior part of the joint below the medial femoral condyle

tissues accommodate themselves to the intruding meniscal fragment by stretching the anterior cruciate ligament, or the development of a groove in the articular cartilage of the femoral condyle.

This type of tear is surprisingly easy to miss at arthroscopy, partly because the fragment may be concealed by synovium in the notch, and partly because it is possible to slip the arthroscope under the fragment and so miss it entirely. If an apparently intact meniscus seems to be unusually narrow and manipulation of the arthroscope unexpectedly difficult, the possibility of a complete bucket handle fragment lying on top of the arthroscope should be considered.

Incomplete (Type II) circumferential tears. The commonest pattern of bucket handle tear

is that in which the anterior extent of the tear falls short of the anterior meniscal insertion, but can still be seen from the antero-lateral approach (Figs. 6.3, 6.4). Meniscal fragments of this type cause locking of the knee with loss of extension, the amount of flexion deformity depending on the thickness of the fragment and the extent of the tear.

Concealed (Type III) circumferential tears. If the anterior limit of the tear cannot be seen from the anterolateral approach because it lies behind the medial femoral condyle (Figs. 6.5, 6.6) there is a real risk that it will be missed. Suspicion that there may be a concealed tear should be aroused if the patient gives a history of definite and dramatic mechanical locking of the knee in full flexion and should be further aroused if the patient is apprehensive when the knee is bent during examination or is unwilling to squat with the knee fully flexed. The preliminary examination under anaesthetic in patients with this type of lesion may demonstrate locking in full flexion, with a marked thud as the fragment is reduced on extension.

At arthroscopy, the meniscus may at first sight seem intact, but on careful observation of its posterior horn as a valgus strain is applied with the tibia externally rotated, a characteristic forward bulging of the meniscus will be seen. The presence of the tear can be confirmed by probing with a percutaneous needle (Figs. 6.7, 6.8) or by traction with a hook inserted from the antero-medial approach (Fig. 6.9).

Partial-thickness posterior horn tears. In this

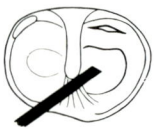

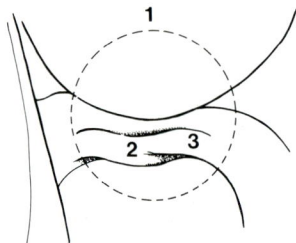

Fig. 6.6 A concealed (Type 3) circumferential tear of the medial meniscus (3) lying in the posterior part of the joint below the medial femoral condyle (1) produce a characteristic forward bulging (2) of the anterior margin of the meniscus

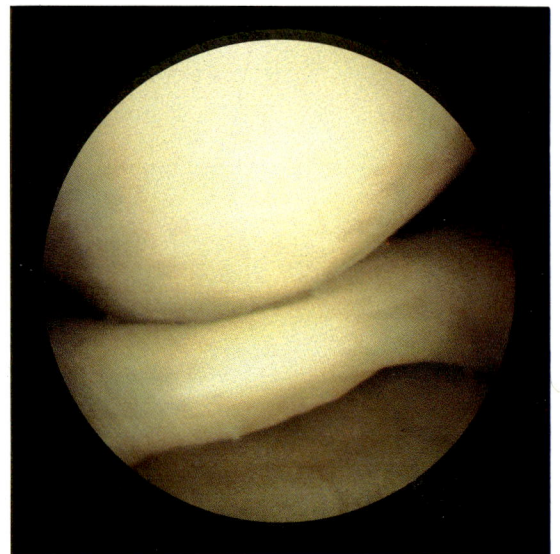

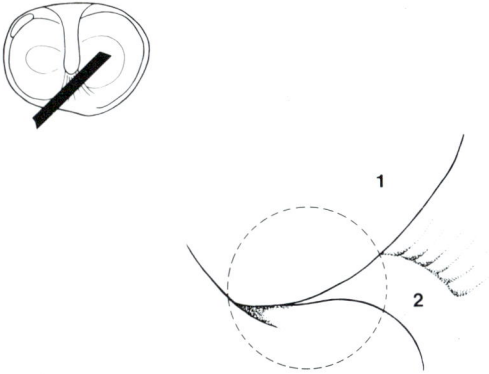

Fig. 6.7 An apparently normal medial meniscus (2) seen from the antero-lateral route (1) medial femoral condyle

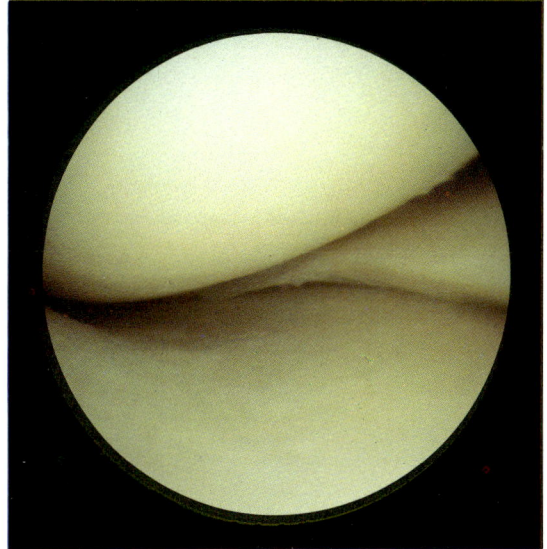

pattern of tear, the split in the meniscus does not extend completely through the meniscus and the blunt hook will demonstrate that although the free edge is abnormally mobile, it is not mobile enough to allow the fragment to come into view in front of the femoral condyle and lie within reach of the operating instruments (Fig. 6.10). These tears are seldom associated with true locking, but may be the cause of pain and discomfort arising from abnormal stretching of the capsule and synovium, and probably progress to a complete tear if left untreated.

Posterior menisco-synovial detachments. Posterior separation of the meniscus is due to a lesion of the coronary ligament of the posterior third of the meniscus rather than the meniscus itself, and is an incomplete form of the peripheral detachment usually found in association with anterior cruciate ligament injuries (Fig. 6.11). This tear is only seen if the postero-medial compartment of the knee can be entered through the notch or from the postero-medial insertion, and even then may be visible only if the meniscus is probed with a hook or needle or if the

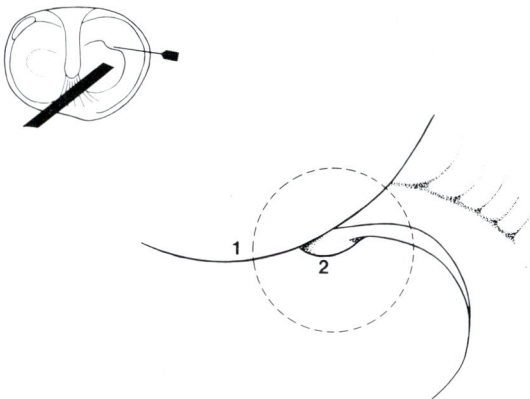

Fig. 6.8 The meniscus illustrated in Figure 6.7, using a percutaneous needle to demonstrate a tear of the inferior surface of the medial meniscus (2)—(1) medial femoral condyle

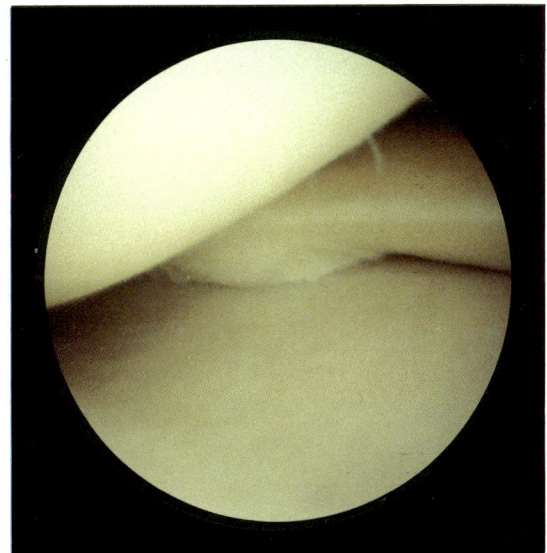

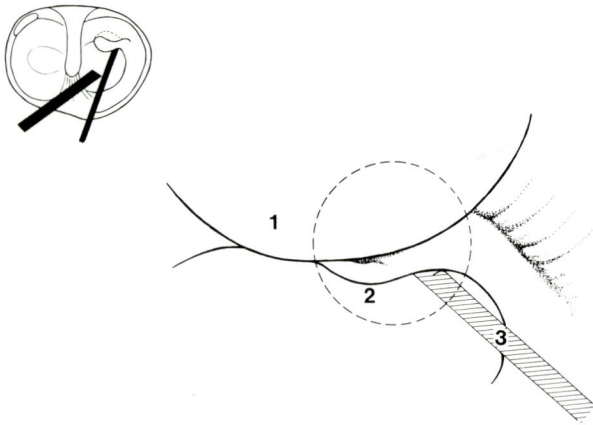

Fig. 6.9 A flap tear of the medial meniscus (2) is pulled from beneath the medial femoral condyle (1) using a blunt hook (3)

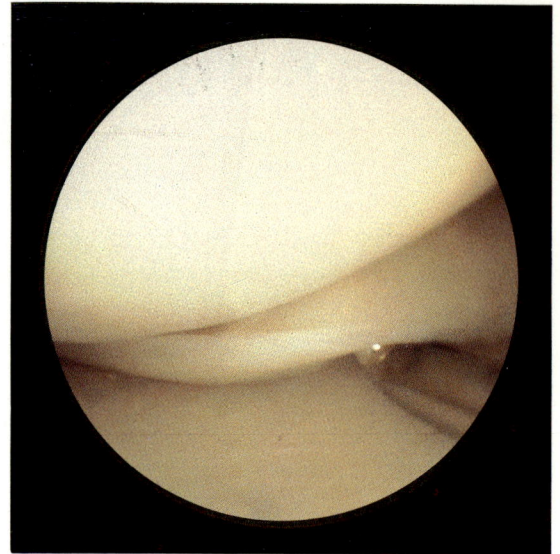

joint is maximally distended with saline under pressure. This type of tear can be treated by either excision of the mobile segment or by reattachment of the meniscus (meniscoresis), but no long-term study is yet available to compare the results of these two techniques.

Detached bucket handle fragments (type IV). Fragments resulting from circumferential tears can become detached at their posterior end to form a large pedunculated tag attached anteriorly (Fig. 6.12). In the medial compartment, bucket handle fragments seldom become detached anteriorly, although this does occur in the lateral compartment. These pedunculated meniscal fragments usually come to lie in the medial gutter where they can be felt as a 'loose body' on clinical examination, but can easily be distin-

guished from a true loose body because they cannot be made to leave the medial gutter. The length of the fragment varies according to the anatomy of the tear from which it arose, the fragments being longer the

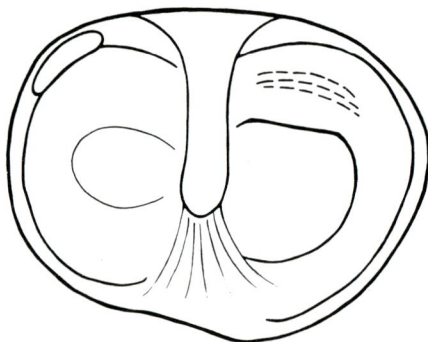

Fig. 6.11 Posterior menisco-synovial detachment in which the meniscus has become detached from the tibia but is itself intact

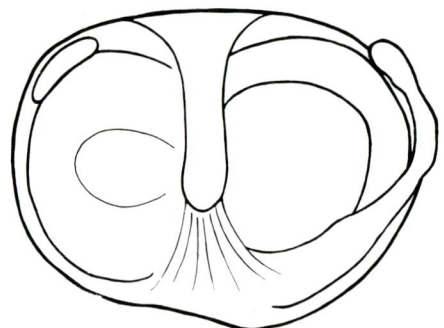

Fig. 6.10 Partial thickness tear of the posterior third of the medial meniscus, which is usually detectable by an abnormal forward protrusion of the posterior edge of the meniscus

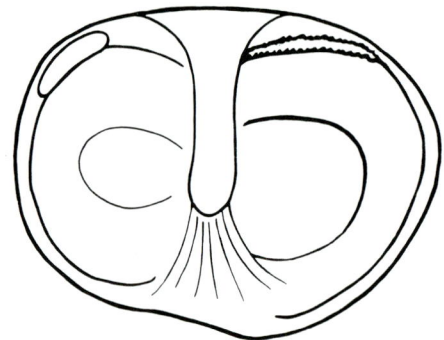

Fig. 6.12 Bucket handle fragment of meniscus which has become detached posteriorly and come to lie in the medial gutter

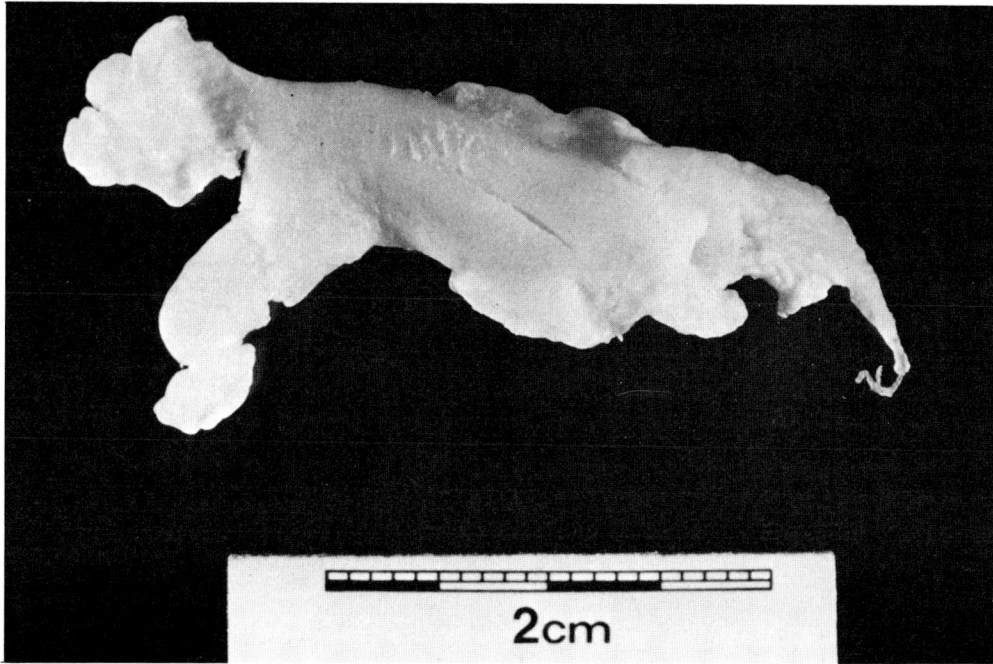

Fig. 6.13 Long detached bucket handle fragment. The free end of the fragment (on the left) has become rounded

further forward the tear extends (Figs. 6.13, 6.14, 6.15, 6.16). Double and triple fragments of this type are sometimes seen (Fig. 6.17).

Detached bucket handle fragments are easily seen at arthroscopy, although those arising in the posterior half of the joint may need to be lifted out of the gutter with a percutaneous needle before the exact anatomy can be demonstrated. The end and the free edges of the fragment are usually smooth and rounded and the fragments are thicker and longer than flaps arising from horizontal tears.

Removing the fragment

Once the anatomy has been defined, the removal of the fragment is comparatively easy. Several methods are available and each will be described.

Double puncture technique.

1. *Type I tears.* These are dealt with by the double puncture technique with operating instruments inserted at the medial edge of the patellar tendon, 1 cm above the meniscus (Fig. 2.9). The fragment should be dislocated into the notch if it is not already there and the posterior attachment divided first with scissors or a knife. The operating scissors are the instrument of choice and will cut the posterior attachment easily if a blade is slipped between the femoral condyle and

the fragment into the 'axilla' of the tear (Fig. 6.18). The temptation to twist the scissors or to take too large a bite must be resisted if damage to the instrument is to be avoided. If the fragment is unusually thick, it will be easier to divide the posterior attachment with the knife or guillotine than with the scissors, but if a guillotine is used to divide the posterior attachment, the fragment is usually divided

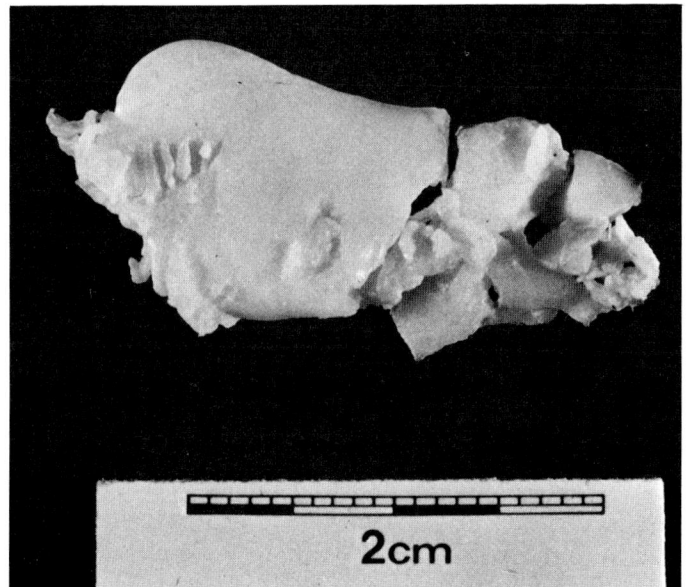

Fig. 6.14 Shorter detached bucket handle fragment. The bulk of the fragment was removed intact and the base trimmed with rongeurs

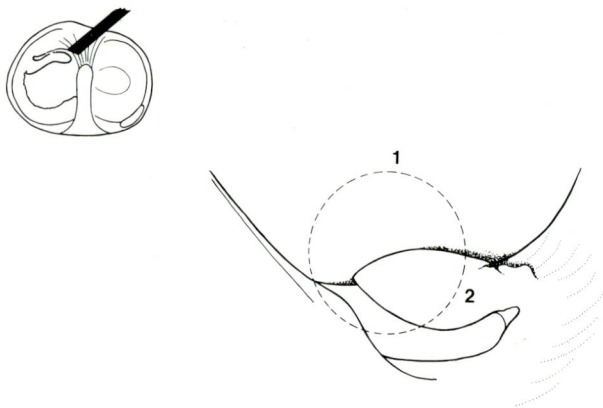

Fig. 6.15 A detached bucket handle fragment of meniscus (2) has come to lie in front of the medial femoral condyle (1) and close to the lens in such a way that it appears larger than its true size

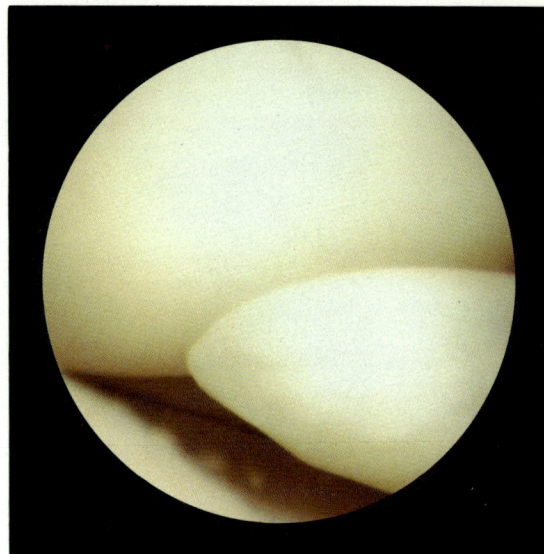

too far anteriorly, leaving a large posterior fragment to be removed piecemeal with punch forceps or pituitary rongeurs.

When the fragment has been divided posteriorly it can be moved away to the medial gutter while the cut posterior attachment is inspected carefully to make certain that there is no retained meniscal fragment (Fig. 6.19). Any stubs of tissue that do remain can be trimmed back with punch forceps or rongeurs, but excessive trimming will damage the meniscal rim and is potentially harmful.

When the fragment has been divided posteriorly, excision can continue in one of two ways. If the operating instrument has been inserted directly above the anterior meniscal attachment, the posterior end of the fragment can be seized with grasping forceps and withdrawn through the skin. The fragment will usually be so large that it will not pass along the instrument cannula, which will be pulled out of the knee by the meniscal fragment. With the fragment protruding through the skin (Fig. 6.20), firm traction can be applied and the anterior attachment divided

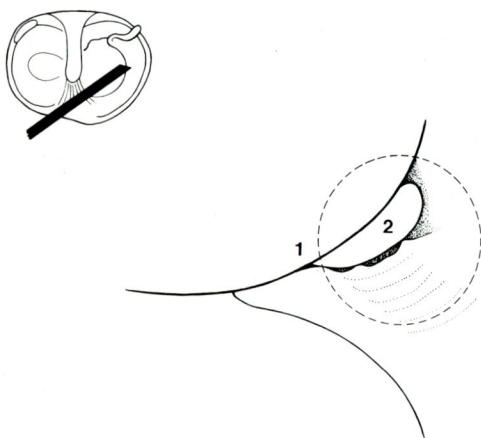

Fig. 6.16 A ruptured bucket handle fragment (2) of medial meniscus which has turned back on itself to lie in the medial gutter beside the medial femoral condyle (1)

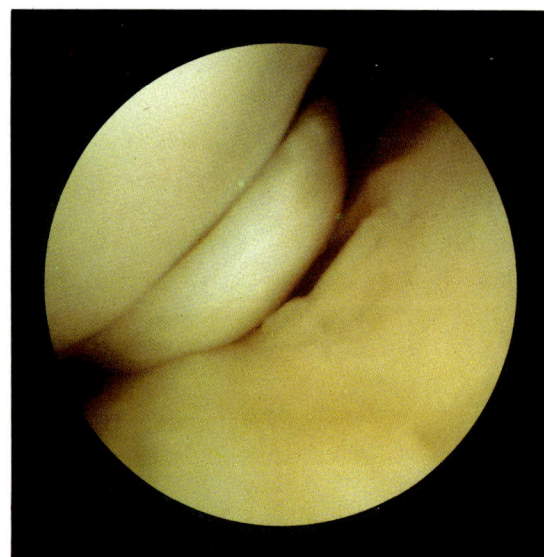

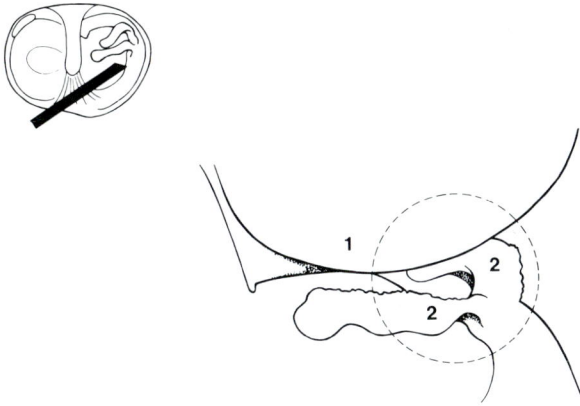

Fig. 6.17 Two detached bucket handle fragments of medial meniscus (2) lying in the medial compartment beneath the medial femoral condyle (1)

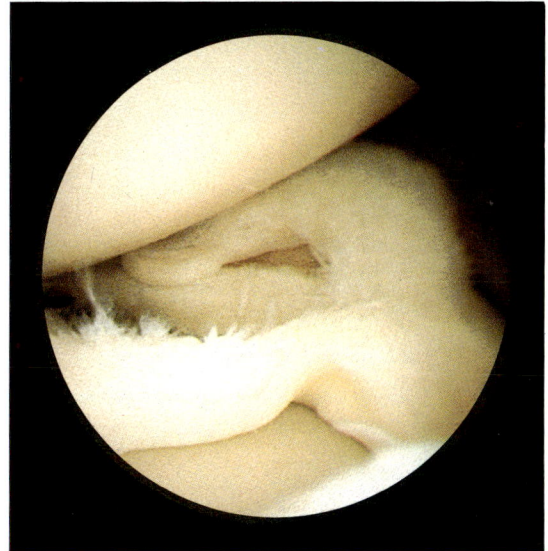

with a No. 15 blade passed through the skin beneath the fragment in such a way that it is divided in the subcutaneous tissues and the fragment removed intact (Fig. 6.21). If the blade is passed above the fragment instead of below, a long anterior tag will remain.

2. Type II tears. Type II fragments and those Type I fragments that cannot be removed by the method described above require a different approach. After dividing the posterior attachment in the manner already described, the anterior attachment is divided

inside the knee before withdrawing the fragment. Operating instruments can usually be brought to bear on the anterior attachment from the antero-medial approach if a valgus and external rotation strain is applied to the knee. Transposition of the instruments from medial to lateral side is seldom necessary, but great care must be taken to manipulate the instruments gently to avoid damaging the articular cartilage.

It is important that the intact meniscal rim is not divided at this stage but this should not occur if the

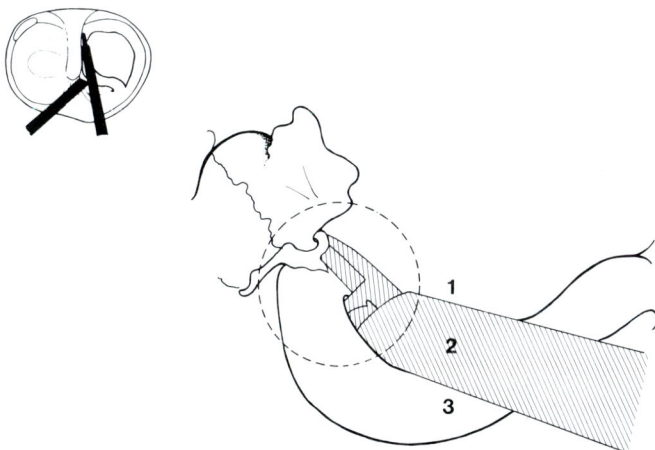

Fig. 6.18 A locked incomplete (Type 2) bucket handle fragment of medial meniscus being divided at its posterior attachment using the arthroscopic scissors (2)—(1) medial femoral condyle

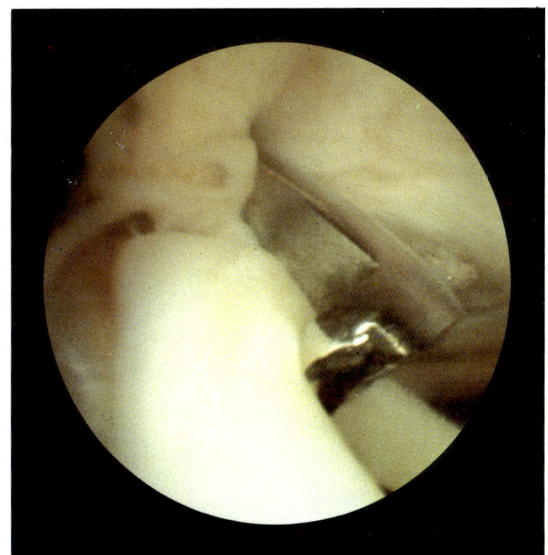

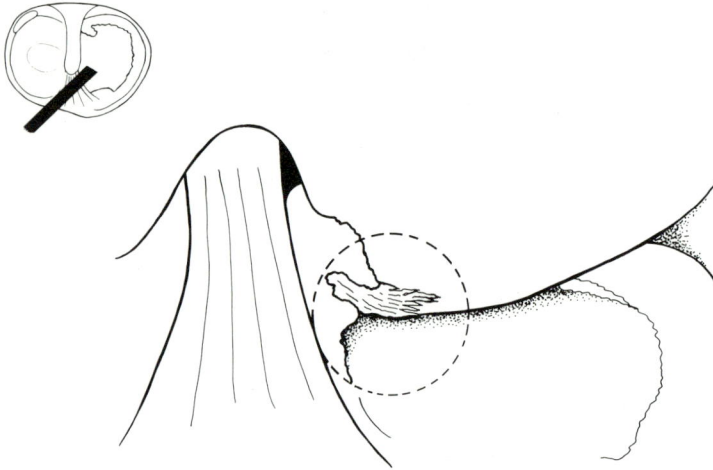

Fig. 6.19 The stump of medial meniscus left after division of its posterior attachment

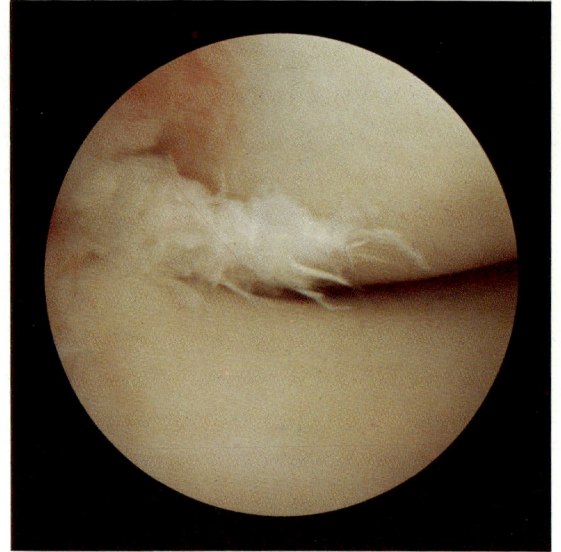

fragment is avulsed or cut with the guillotine. Division of the rim with the knife or scissors makes the rim unstable and can lead to continuing symptoms, which will not be relieved until a total meniscectomy is performed.

The simplest and most effective way to divide the fragment anteriorly is to grasp it firmly at its base with curved or straight rongeurs and avulse it (Fig. 6.22). If the rongeurs are applied correctly, the fragment will come out intact, leaving a smooth base and an intact rim.

An alternative is to divide the anterior attachment with scissors, a knife or a guillotine Fig. 6.23), but complete division of the fragment will leave it free and in danger of floating off as a loose body (Fig. 6.24). This accident can be avoided by grasping the fragment with a second instrument such as tendon forceps inserted through a third channel or by leaving a few strands of meniscal tissue intact so that the fragment can be avulsed with grasping forceps. To judge the amount of meniscal tissue that can be avulsed easily with forceps requires some experience, and attempts to grub out the meniscus by its roots with Kocher's forceps should be avoided. If the attachment is inadvertently divided completely before the fragment has been grasped securely, the 'loose body procedure' described in Chapter 5 should be instituted immediately, and the fragment retrieved as soon as possible.

Some surgeons prefer to divide the anterior attach-

ment before the posterior. Although the anterior attachment is the easier of the two to divide, division of the anterior attachment brings the very real danger that the meniscal fragment will drop back into the postero-medial compartment (Fig. 6.25) making retrieval difficult. If the fragment should escape in this way, it can be fished out of the postero-medial compartment with a blunt hook inserted from either the antero-medial or central approach, but it can be removed more neatly with curved rongeurs inserted from the postero-medial route under control of the arthroscope passed into the postero-medial compart-

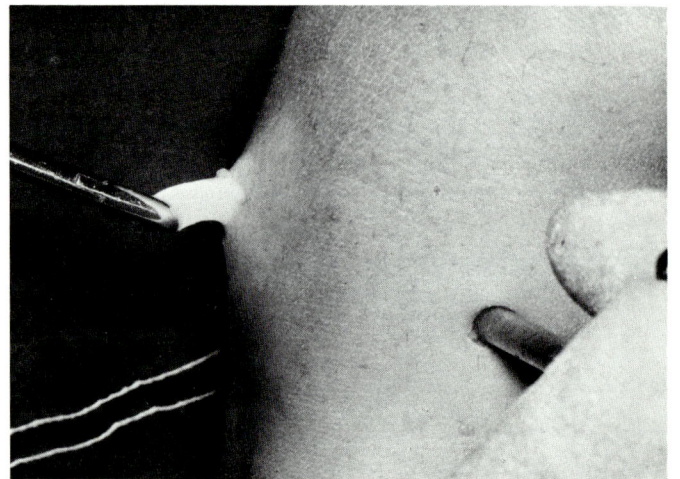

Fig. 6.20 A bucket handle fragment of medial meniscus has been divided posteriorly with arthroscopic scissors and drawn through the skin with pituitary rongeurs

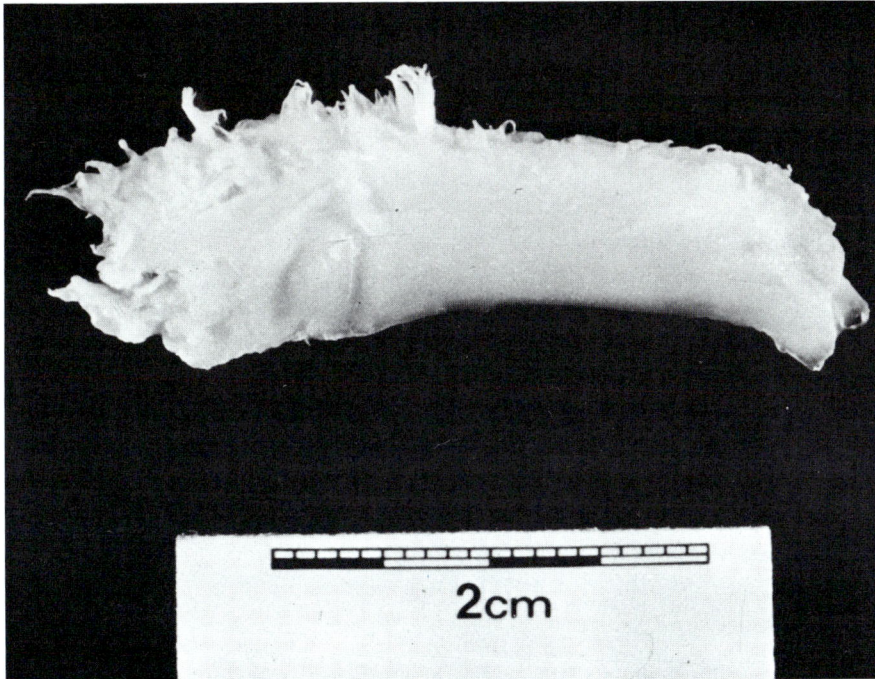

Fig. 6.21 Bucket handle fragment of meniscus removed intact

ment through the intercondylar notch. Alternatively, the arthroscope can be inserted postero-medially and the rongeurs through the notch.

Both of the techniques described above may prove impossible if the fragment is so tightly jammed in the front of the femoral condyle that the blade of the scissors cannot be insinuated between the fragment and the condyle. In these circumstances there are two possible solutions. In the first, the fragment is divided at its centre with the knife, minimising the risk of damage to articular cartilage by leaving a few strands of intact meniscus which can then be ruptured by extending the knee. The two ends of the fragment are then removed piecemeal (Fig. 6.26), a tedious and sometimes untidy procedure. Alternatively, if access is difficult with the fragment dislocated in front of the

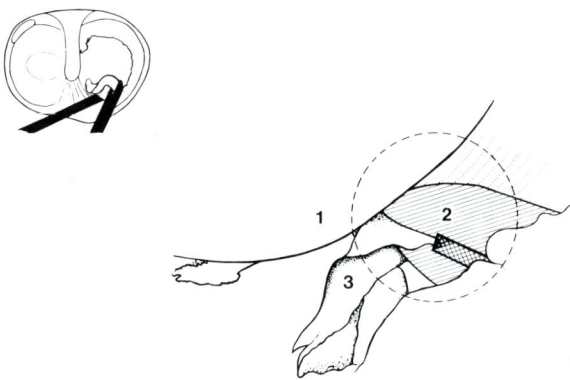

Fig. 6.22 Having divided a bucket handle fragment of medial meniscus posteriorly, the fragment (3) is grasped with pituitary rongeurs (2) at its anterior attachment—(1) medial femoral condyle

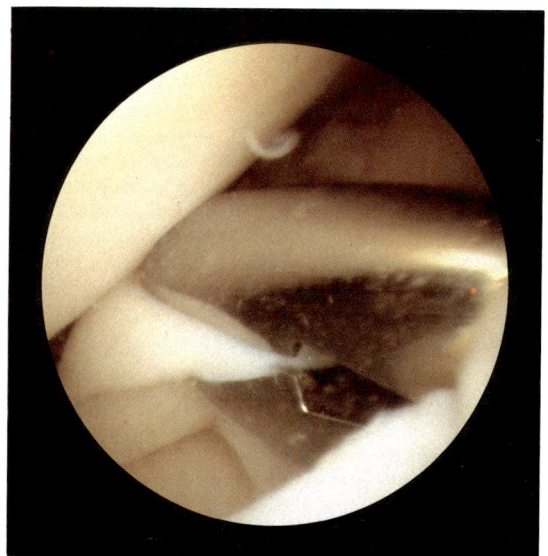

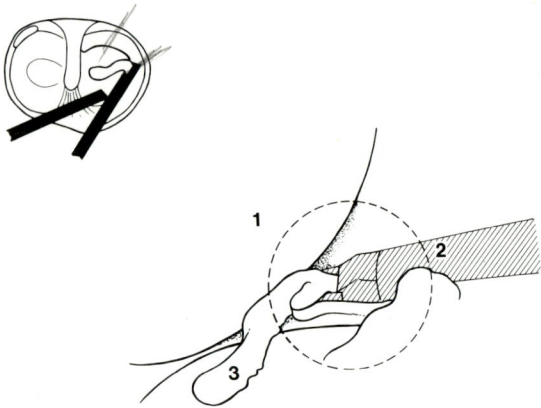

Fig. 6.23 a detached bucket handle fragment of medial meniscus (3) is divided with the arthroscopic guillotine (2) as it lies beneath the medial femoral condyle (1)

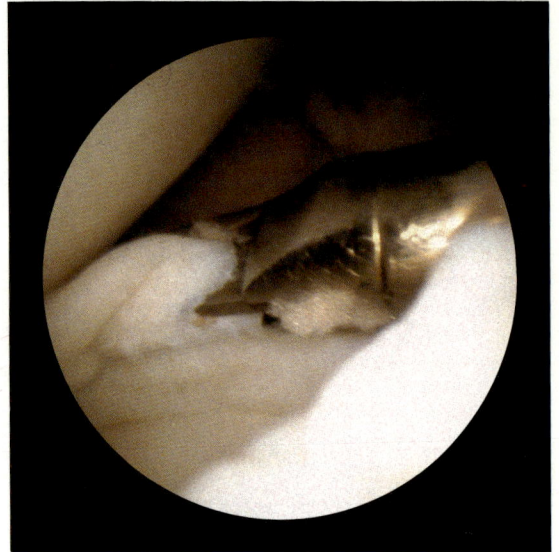

condyle, reduction may simplify the problem but special care must be taken to ensure that the loose fragment is redislocated after division of its anterior attachment, and removed completely. If this precaution is not taken, a large fragment of meniscus will be left in the knee.

3. *Type III tears and menisco-synovial separations.* Dealing with concealed (Type III) fragments and posterior third menisco-synovial separations presents some technical problems whatever technique is used.

Neither end of the tear is visible with the arthroscope, and the tear lies in the least accessible area of the knee. The fragment cannot be dislocated by full flexion with the arthroscope in the joint, and the postero-medial approach is unhelpful except for confirmation of the diagnosis. These problems can be reduced but not abolished by accurate placement of the arthroscope and the instruments, and by correct manipulation of the knee. The instruments should be inserted immediately above the anterior horn of the meniscus about

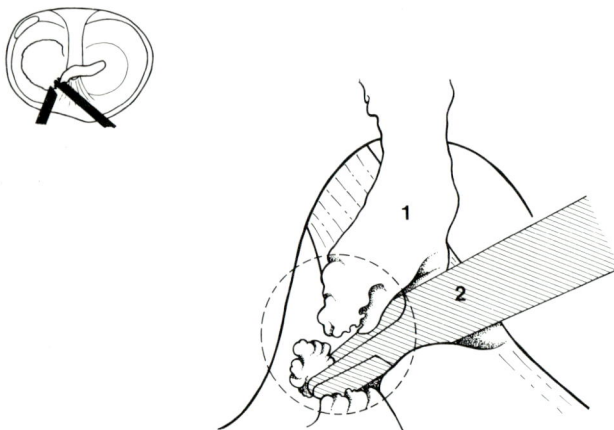

Fig. 6.24 A lateral meniscal fragment (1), having been detached posteriorly, is then detached anteriorly with the punch scissors (2) to create a loose body which floated off to the postero-medial compartment and proved difficult to remove

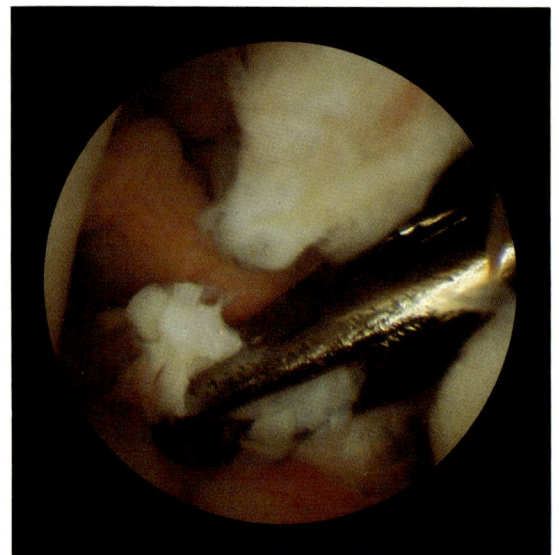

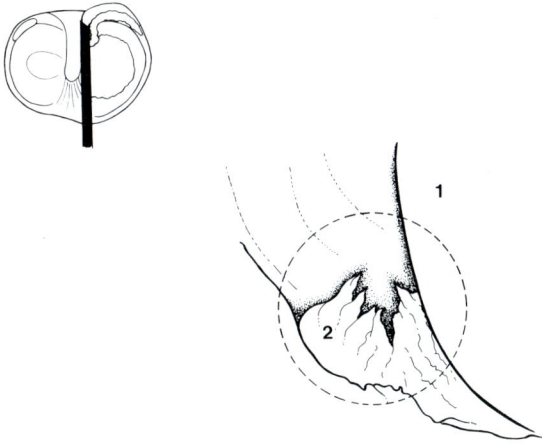

Fig. 6.25 A large fragment of medial meniscus (2) lying in the postero-medial compartment behind the medial femoral condyle (1)

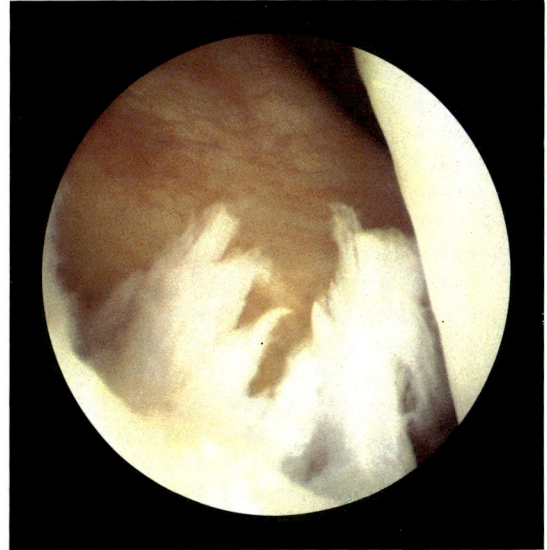

1 cm medial to the edge of the patellar tendon so that they lie flat on the tibial plateau (Fig. 2.9). The blunt hook can then be slipped under the meniscus just in front of the femoral condyle and slid sideways behind the condyle to the site of the tear. If the hook is then turned so that its tip lies against the under-surface of the meniscus, it can be used to pull the fragment forward. When using hooks in this way, they must be turned so that the tip of the hook trails behind the shaft of the instrument as described in Chapter 3; attempts to move the hook with the tip leading will damage the instrument, as well as structures in the joint.

When the tip of the hook is engaged on the under-surface of the posterior horn of the meniscus a strong valgus and external rotation force should be applied to the tibia, and the hook used to draw the loose segment of meniscus in front of the femoral condyle so that its full extent can be appreciated. The fragment will usually remain in the dislocated position where it can either be divided at its posterior and anterior attachments or removed piecemeal, but if it slips back under the femoral condyle, the guillotine, scissors or punch forceps can be passed to the site of its anterior attachment which can then be divided so that the segment is freed and comes to lie in the intercondylar notch. Because fragments resulting from this type of tear are seldom more than 1.5 cm in length, they do not tend to fall back into the posterior compartment. These fragments cannot be reached with instruments passed directly across the joint between tibial and femoral condyles unless the joint is unusually lax and attempts to remove fragments in this way can only result in damage to articular cartilage.

4. *Detached bucket handle fragments.* These fragments can be regarded as bucket handle fragments in which the posterior attachment has already been divided and may be avulsed with rongeurs or divided at their base with a guillotine inserted from the antero-medial route immediately above the medial meniscus and approximately 1 cm from the medial edge of the patellar ligament. If the guillotine or scissors are used rather than rongeurs, even more care must be taken than usual to prevent the fragment escaping and becoming a true loose body because its smooth surface and rounded edges make it unusually mobile and elusive. A percutaneous needle, grasping forceps or tendon forceps can be used to tether the fragment before its base is divided to prevent this difficulty.

5. *Partial thickness tears.* Excision of mobile fragments arising from partial thickness posterior third tears is even more difficult because the fragment cannot be brought within range of the operating instruments, but a combination of traction with the blunt hook and avulsion with curved rongeurs will be successful in removing all abnormally mobile tissues. Any meniscal tissue that cannot be manipulated into the centre of the joint with the percutaneous needle or probing hook is best left where it lies and the operation considered complete when all abnormally mobile

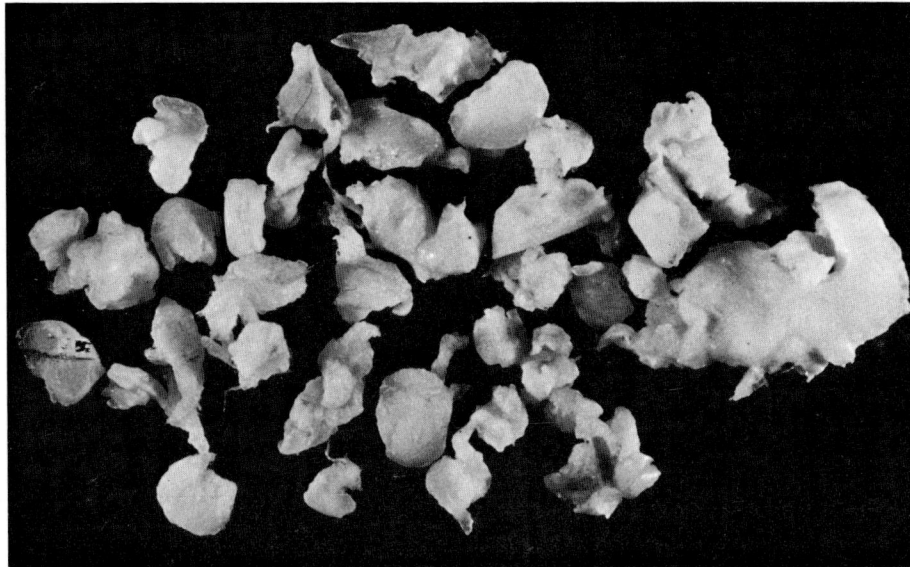

(a)

Fig. 6.26 (a) fragments of meniscus removed piecemeal and (b) reassembled to demonstrate the volume of meniscus removed

(b)

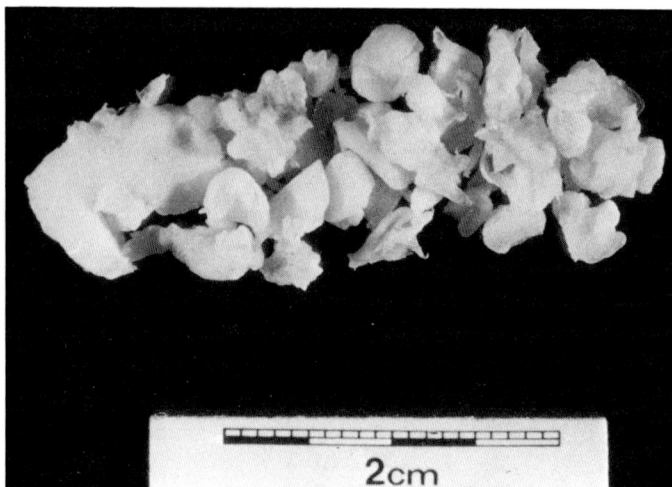

2cm

tissue has been removed and the hook demonstrates only an intact and stable rim.

Using the operating arthroscope. Some surgeons, notably Dr R L O'Connor and Dr R Metcalf, prefer to use the operating arthroscope for the excision of some meniscal fragments. To remove a bucket handle fragment, the diagnostic arthroscope is removed from the antero-lateral approach and the operating arthroscope inserted from the antero-medial approach. The fragment is then seized with grasping forceps or tendon forceps inserted from the antero-lateral approach, and slight tension applied to the fragment by an assistant. The anterior attachment is then divided with the scissors of the operating

arthroscope. Because the fragment is securely held it cannot fall back into the postero-medial compartment, and can be lifted with slight tension so that the posterior attachment can also be divided with the scissors of the operating arthroscope.

This technique is effective, but requires considerable skill with the operating arthroscope. There is also the risk that excessive traction will be applied to the fragment so that the division of its base extends more deeply into the substance of the meniscus than did the original tear. Apart from these technical difficulties, there is the practical problem that the scissors and basket forceps have a short working life and need frequent replacement.

Triple puncture technique. When the central approach is used for diagnostic arthroscopy, the arthroscope can be left *in situ* throughout the procedure and instruments brought to bear upon the lesion from both antero-medial and antero-lateral approaches. The control of three instruments is more difficult than two, but the technique has the great virtue that large instruments can be used to cut the meniscus from the side instead of relying upon the more delicate instruments of the operating arthroscope which can only be moved parallel with the telescope itself.

The first step in the removal of a locked bucket handle fragment using the triple puncture technique should be to grasp the fragment with forceps inserted from the antero-lateral route. A knife inserted from

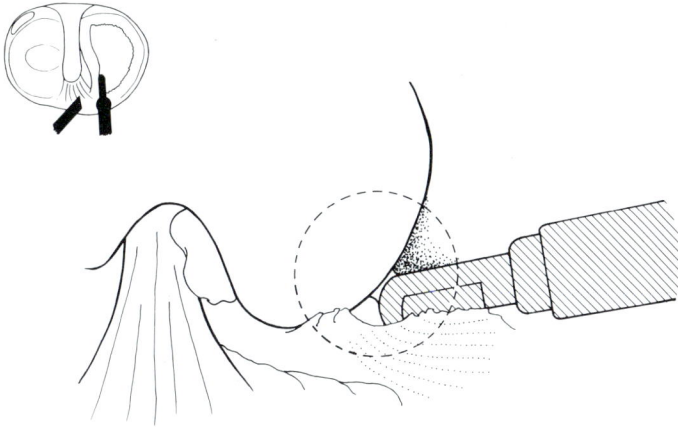

Fig. 6.27 Dividing the anterior attachment of a locked bucket handle fragment of meniscus using the central approach for the triple puncture technique

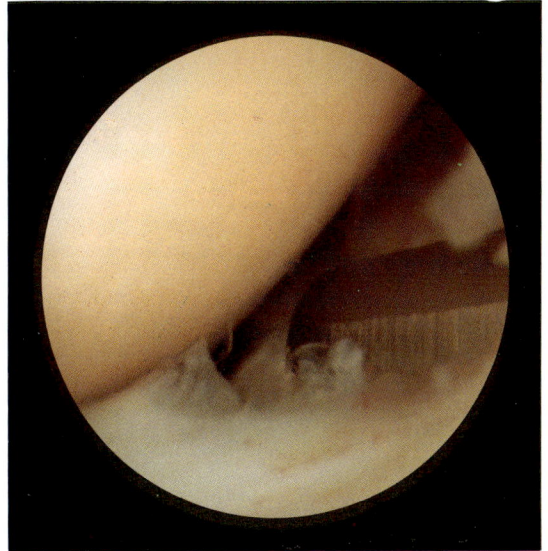

the antero-medial route can then be used to divide the anterior attachment while gentle traction is applied with the grasping forceps (Fig. 6.27). The fragment of meniscus, now detached anteriorly, is held with the grasping forceps (Fig. 6.28) to prevent it escaping into the postero-medial compartment and is divided at its posterior attachment with the knife inserted from the antero-medial route while gentle traction is applied (Fig. 6.29). The fragment is sometimes easier to manage, and to divide, if it is first twisted with the

grasping forceps. If the use of two instruments as well as the arthroscope is necessary and the surgeon does not wish to violate the patellar tendon, the instruments can be manipulated under the control of the arthroscope inserted from the lateral midpatellar approach, as suggested by Dr D Patel (Fig. 6.30).

The differences between these techniques is slight and should not become either a preoccupation or bone of contention amoung those who practise arthroscopic surgery.

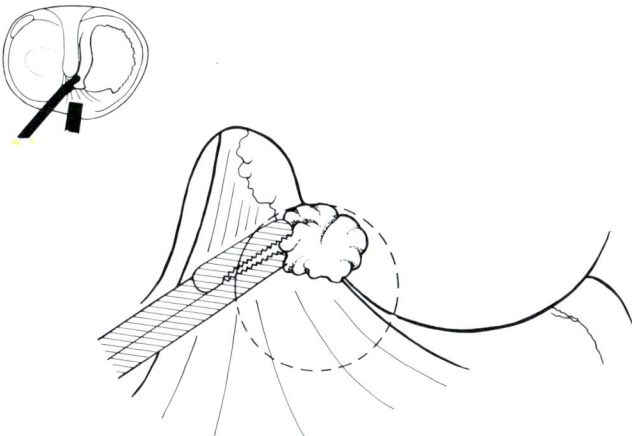

Fig. 6.28 The bucket handle fragment of meniscus illustrated in Figure 6.27 after division of its anterior attachment. The fragment is grasped with tendon tunnelling forceps

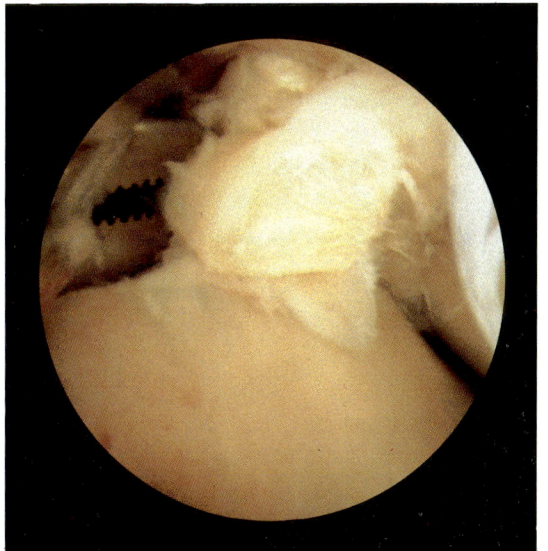

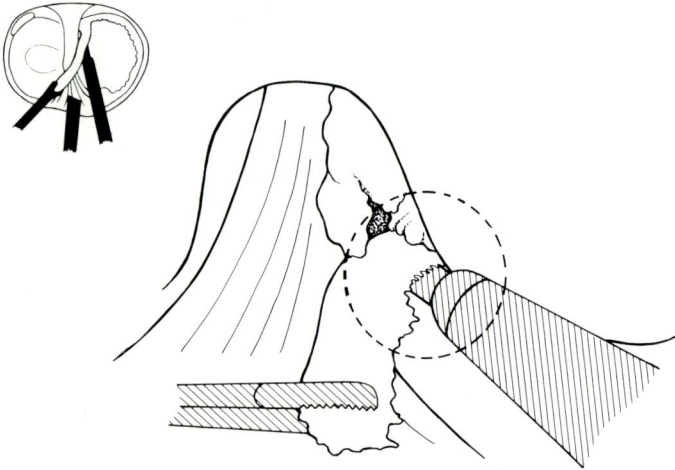

Fig. 6.29 Dividing the posterior attachment of the fragment illustrated in Figure 6.27 and 6.28 while traction is applied with the tendon tunnelling forceps

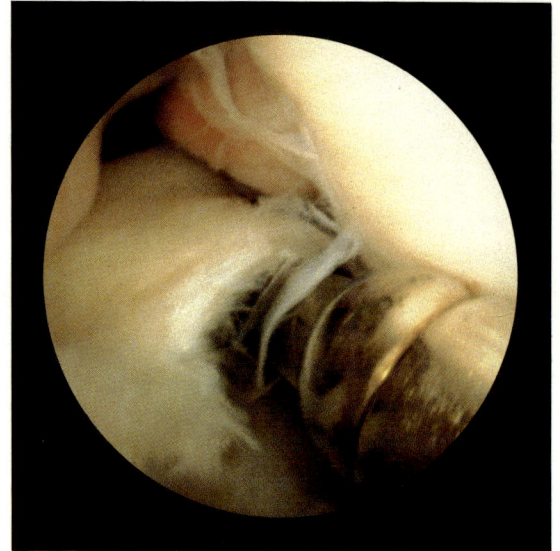

Powered instrument technique. The use of the meniscus cutter is advised by some, but it is not as effective as might be hoped. The meniscus has a grain formed by the parallel fibres that make up its substance, and it is easier to follow the grain of the meniscus with hand operated instruments than powered cutters. The powered cutter is most effective for removing flaps that are small enough to be drawn into the mouth of the instrument, but is less effective for cutting across the grain of a bucket handle fragment. The powered shaver, if it is to be used, should be used in conjunction with other instruments and not instead of them, and is perhaps at its most useful in the trimming of an irregular meniscal rim (Fig. 6.50).

Although the meniscus cutter is effective when

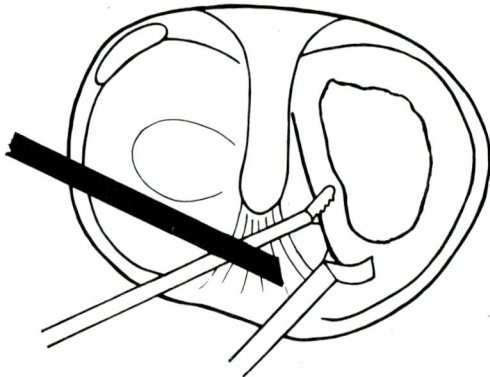

Fig. 6.30 The triple puncture technique with the arthroscope inserted from the lateral midpatellar route

cutting meniscus, it is even more effective when cutting articular cartilage or synovium and great caution is required in its use. The ideal instrument for removing menisci would be a wand-like tool only one or two millimetres in diameter which would cause meniscal tissue to melt away on contact with its tip. It has not yet been invented.

Total meniscectomy. The techniques so far described deal only with the removal of loose meniscal fragments, but it is also possible to perform a total or sub-total meniscectomy under arthroscopic control. A technique has been developed by Oretorp and Gillquist which depends upon a peripheral incision made with a sharp blade so that the entire meniscus becomes, in effect, a large bucket handle fragment.

The incision is begun anteriorly using a knife inserted from the antero-medial approach and is carried as far back in the medial gutter and as close to the anterior attachment of the meniscus as possible. The arthroscope is then passed through the notch into the postero-medial compartment, and the knife inserted from the postero-medial approach. The posterior limit of the incision is identified and the cut continued laterally to the posterior attachment of the meniscus. The entire meniscus can then either be dislocated in the notch and removed in the same way as any other bucket handle fragment, or the anterior and posterior attachment divided and the meniscus removed though either the antero-medial or postero-medial incisions.

The indications for this procedure are somewhat limited if the principles of conservative meniscal surgery already propounded are followed and are probably confined to the removal of shattered menisci, menisci with totally disrupted rims, and those affected by cystic degeneration.

Despite these limitations, the technique is of great importance if only because it makes arthroscopic meniscectomy available to those surgeons who still prefer total to partial meniscectomy and who would otherwise be unable to find a place in their practice either for the arthroscope or for arthroscopic surgery.

Flaps

Flap tears arising from horizontal fissures in the posterior third of the meniscus must be distinguished from detached bucket handle fragments. Detached bucket handle fragments are thicker than true flap tears, generally occur in younger patients, and can be avulsed to leave a firm and even rim while horizontal flaps are more common in older patients and leave an irregular meniscal surface.

Superior flaps. Flaps arising from the upper surface of the meniscus (Fig. 6.31) or its free margin, and based anteriorly at the junction of the middle and posterior thirds of the meniscus, are the easiest to remove. Flaps of this type are usually associated with a sensation of catching or instability in the postero-medial part of the joint rather than true locking and

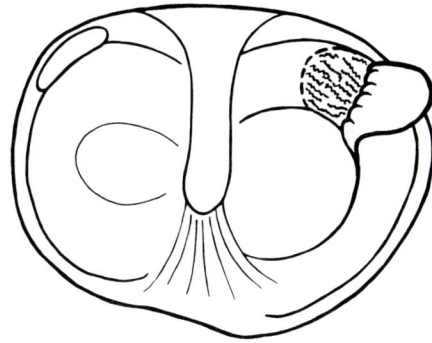

Fig. 6.31 A flap of tissue raised from the superior surface of the medial meniscus

the symptoms are dramatically relieved by the removal of the offending flap, which is usually the size of a little finger nail and involves the upper surface of the meniscus only. These flaps may be inconspicuous at arthroscopy, but are well-demonstrated with the blunt hook or needle or simply by a valgus and external rotation force (Figs. 6.32, 6.33). Occasionally, the flaps become tucked beneath the meniscus where they present the appearance of an inferior flap and may be suspected only because of an unusually smooth and rounded margin to the meniscus. If the margin of the meniscus appears round rather than sharp in its posterior third, a flap tear of this type should always be considered.

Inferior flaps. Flaps arising from the under-surface of the medial meniscus are rarer than those arising from the upper surface (Fig. 6.34). As with

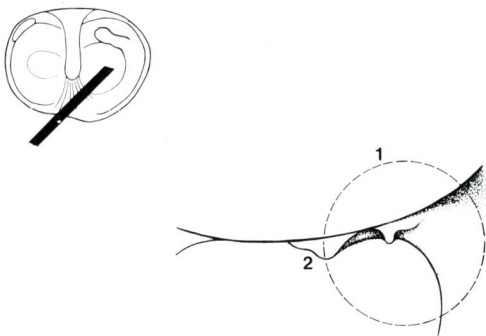

Fig. 6.32 A flap of medial meniscus just visible below the medial femoral condyle (1)—(2) medial tibial plateau

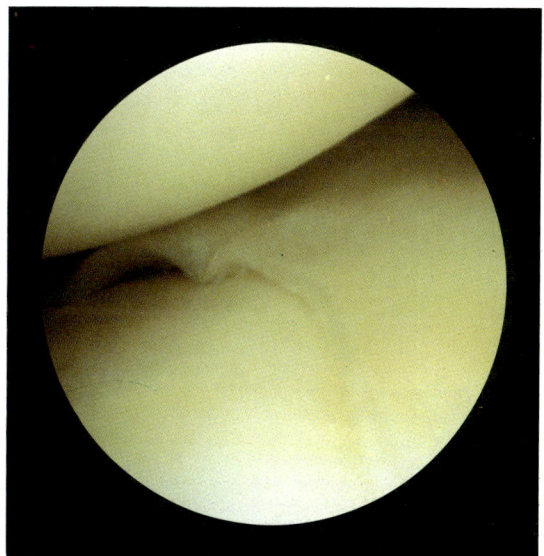

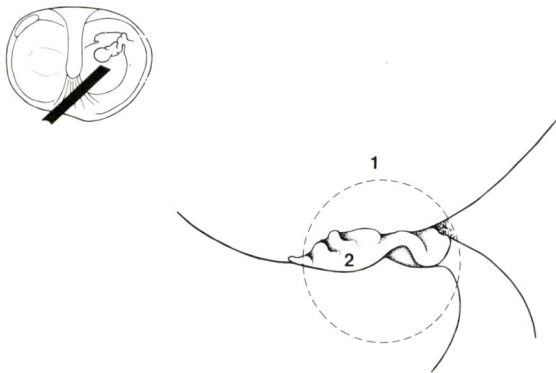

Fig. 6.33 The flap shown in Figure 6.32 (2) is manipulated from beneath the medial femoral condyle (1) by a valgus and external rotation force

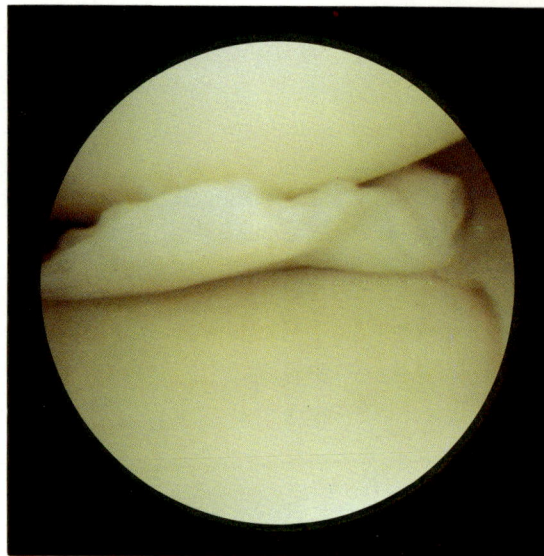

other lesions of the posterior third of the meniscus, inferior flaps are easily missed and are sometimes found only with the help of a percutaneous needle sweeping beneath the meniscus (Fig. 6.35). The presence of a posterior third flap should be suspected on clinical grounds if the patient complains of a 'catching' in the medial side of the joint or if there is a constant click arising from the postero-medial compartment on rotation and flexion.

Degenerate flaps. The flaps described above

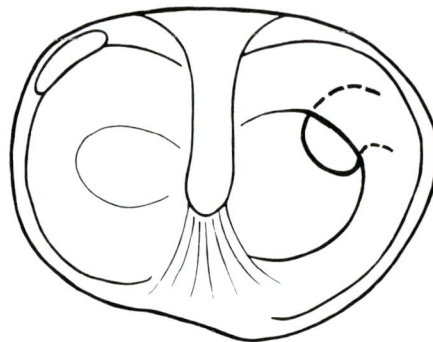

Fig. 6.34 A flap arising from the inferior surface of the medial meniscus

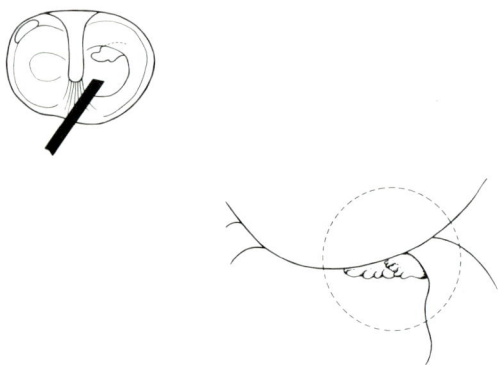

Fig. 6.35 A flap of meniscal tissue arising from the inferior surface of the posterior horn of the medial meniscus

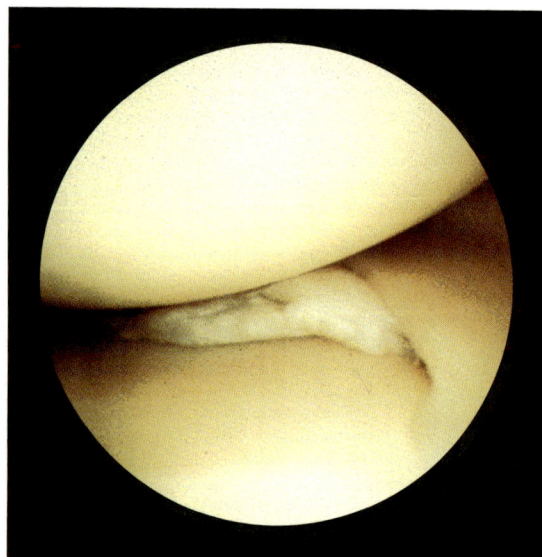

consist of relatively healthy meniscal tissue with a smooth upper surface and an irregular lower surface, but tears are sometimes found which consist of nothing more than a mass of fluffy degenerate tissue (Figs. 6.36, 6.37) arising from either the upper or lower surfaces of the meniscus. These tears are most common in older patients with degenerative joint disease.

Shattered meniscus. Some menisci present so many splits and tears that the lesion cannot be assigned to any one of the categories mentioned and appear as a mass of shredded meniscal tissue (Figs. 6.38, 6.39) all of which must be removed. Shattered menisci are most commonly seen in patients with ruptured anterior cruciate ligaments and gross ligamentous instability.

Removing the fragment

Double puncture technique. Flaps are best removed by avulsion with forceps or rongeurs applied to their base or by division of the base with scissors. Curved rongeurs are a little large for this procedure but have the advantage that they can be slipped easily around the medial gutter at the base of the flap, and fine punch forceps are also suitable if the blade can be slipped under the flap (Figs. 6.40, 6.41). Fluffy degenerate flaps are usually too soft to be avulsed neatly, and must be picked off with fine basket forceps. The surgeon must accept that it is not possible to

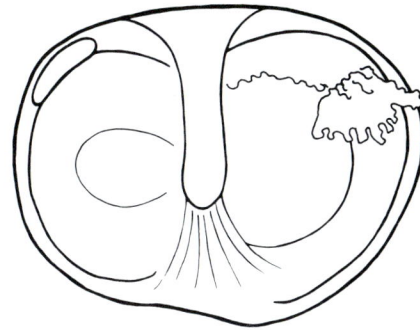

Fig. 6.36 A flap of fluffy degenerative meniscus arising from the superior surface

achieve arthroscopic cosmesis after excision of this type of tear.

Inferior flaps can be avulsed with basket forceps or rongeurs, but tend to fall back under the meniscus before it can be grasped. The percutaneous needle can be used to hold the flap forwards so that it can be seized with forceps, but care must be taken not to remove the tip of the needle as well as the flap.

There is no simple answer to the problem of the completely shattered meniscus, which must either be removed piece by piece with rongeurs and punch forceps until the percutaneous needle and hook reveal an intact, stable rim, or excised using the technique for total meniscectomy described above (p. ooo).

Operating arthroscope. The operating arthroscope can be used to remove meniscal flaps. The same principles are followed as for bucket handle tears,

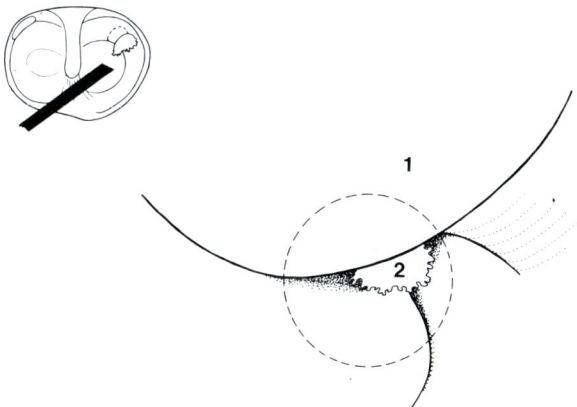

Fig. 6.37 A flap of degenerate meniscal tissue (2) arising from the upper surface of the meniscus has fallen forwards to lie beneath the medial femoral condyle

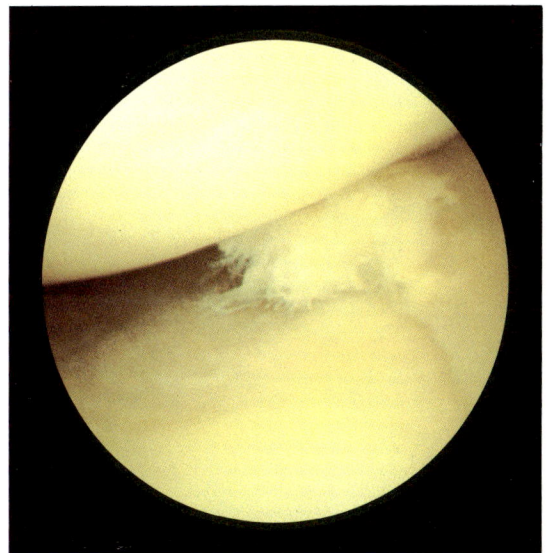

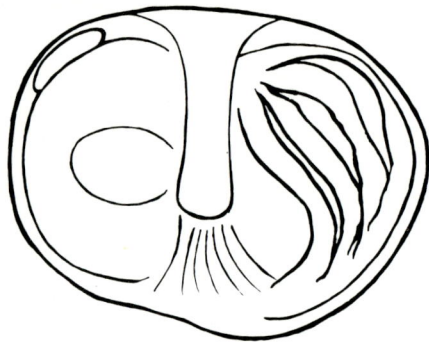

Fig. 6.38 A completely shattered medial meniscus

tension being applied to the flap with forceps inserted from the lateral compartment so that the flap can be cut neatly at its base with the scissors of the operating arthroscope inserted from the antero-medial approach (Figs. 6.42, 6.43).

This technique is effective, but as with removal of bucket handle fragments, requires skill in the handling of the operating arthroscope and the insertion of three instruments rather than two.

Triple puncture technique. The triple puncture technique can be used for the removal of flaps but it may be difficult to see the posterior third of the meniscus from the central or lateral suprapatellar approach and this technique is less effective for the removal of flaps than for the removal of bucket handle fragments, although it is invaluable if the flap is long and its base difficult to reach without the help of traction (Fig. 6.44).

The degenerate posterior horn

When degenerate osteoarthritis is present, the meniscus usually shares in the degenerative process and assessment of the meniscus should concentrate on the stability of the rim rather than the smoothness of its surface (Figs. 6.45, 6.46). Attempts to remove small flaps or loose strands of meniscal tissue can be a thankless task that may cause the surgeon to wish that he had not become involved. As one small irregularity is removed, two more may appear and repeated use of the operating instruments in the posterior part of the joint is likely to damage the femoral condyle and do more harm than good. The surgeon should therefore confine himself to removing only unstable flaps or tags which can be dealt with according to the methods already described, and avoid excessive zeal.

Retained posterior horn fragments

If a patient's symptoms persist after a meniscectomy done without a preliminary arthroscopy or arthrogram, it is likely that meniscectomy was the wrong operation. A review of patients with persistent symptoms after meniscectomy (Dandy and Jackson, 1976) showed that retained fragments were rare, and that the commonest abnormality associated with persistent symptoms after meniscectomy was degenerative arthritis. In the days before arthroscopy, the 'retained fragment' offered a convenient explanation for failure after partial meniscectomy, with the result

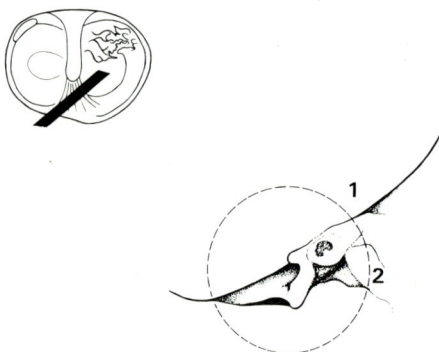

Fig. 6.39 A completely shattered medial meniscus (2) without any intact rim—(1) medial femoral condyle

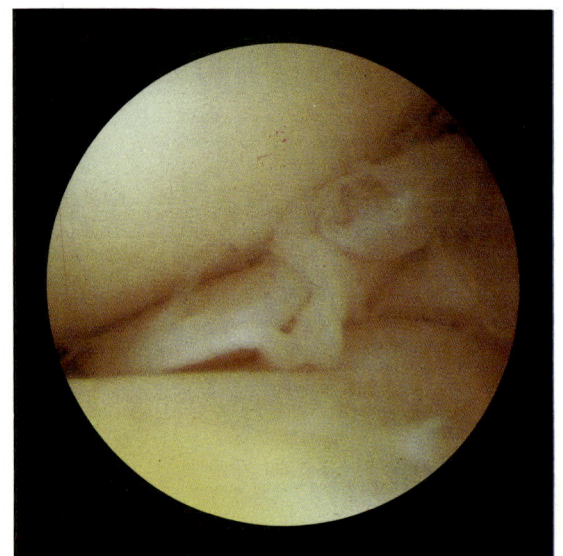

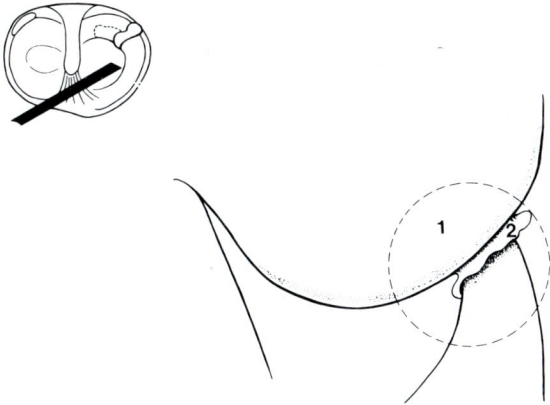

Fig. 6.40 A flap of meniscal tissue involving the upper surface of the meniscus only (2) has come forward beneath the medial femoral condyle (1) to lie in the medial gutter

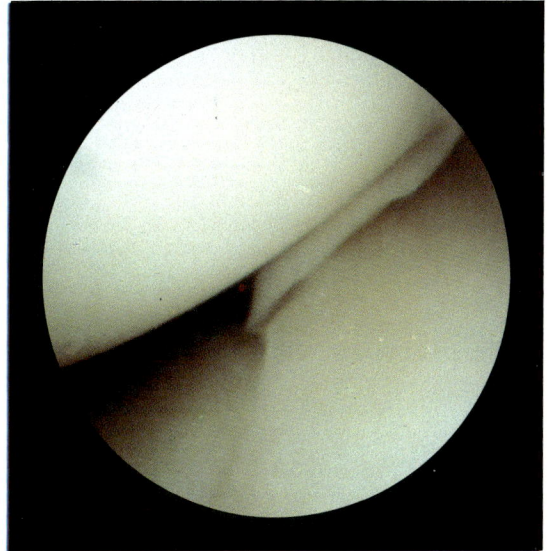

that partial meniscectomy itself often became the scapegoat for a wrong initial diagnosis.

The open removal of retained fragments of posterior horn can be a tedious procedure involving a wide arthrotomy and yielding little more than a tatty scrap of tissue so firmly adherent to the bone that its excision is difficult and it relationship to the patient's symptoms obscure. It is not surprising that the clinical results of excision of retained fragments of posterior horn are unimpressive.

Despite these comments, retained fragments of posterior horn do occur occasionally, and can easily be retrieved arthroscopically. The presence of a fragment can be confirmed by passing the arthroscope into the postero-medial compartment through the notch or the postero-medial approach, if necessary using a blunt hook to explore the posterior attachment of the meniscus. The fragment can then be drawn forwards into the notch from which it can be removed piecemeal with punch forceps or rongeurs in the same way as the

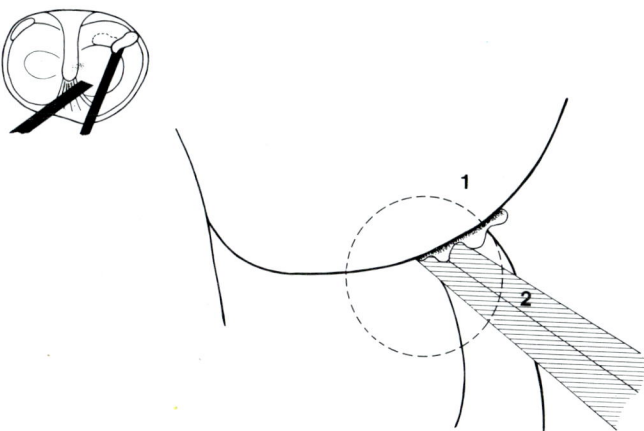

Fig. 6.41 The meniscal flap illustrated in Figure 6.40 is divided at its base with fine punch scissors (2) slipped beneath the meniscus and the medial femoral condyle (1)

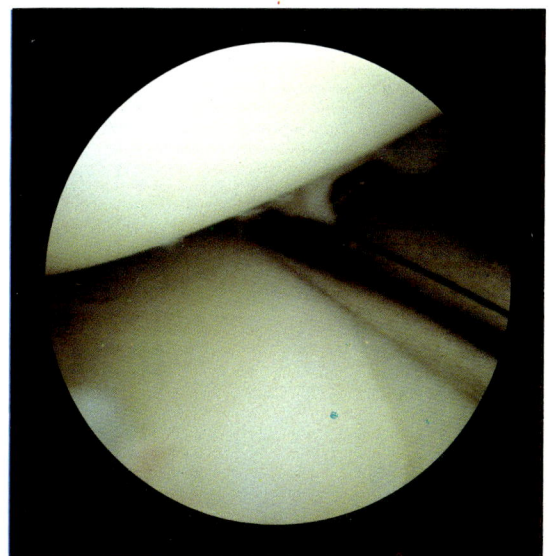

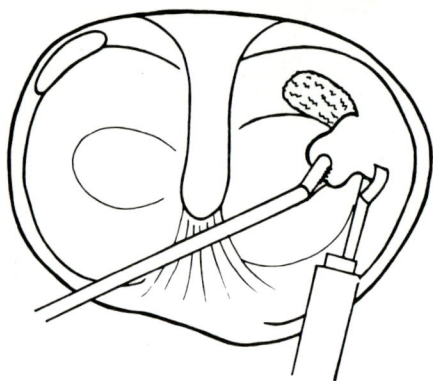

Fig. 6.42 Using the operating arthroscope to remove a flap of tissue while traction is applied with forceps inserted from the antero-lateral route

posterior end of bucket handle fragment. Alternatively, curved pituitary rongeurs inserted from the postero-medial approach can be used to remove it from behind.

Checking the rim

When the fragment has been removed, the rim can be trimmed with precision using punch forceps or rongeurs. To know when the rim has been trimmed sufficiently requires considerable judgement and it is for this reason that the author regards it as the most difficult stage of the operation.

If the fragment is particularly thick, the step at the anterior extent of the meniscal tear will be difficult to remove completely (Fig. 6.47) but can be relied upon to round off further with the passage of time (Fig.

6.48). When trimming is completed, the rim must again be examined carefully with the probing hook in the usual way to make certain that it is still stable (Fig. 6.49). Excessive trimming of the rim can result in needless damage to the intact and stable meniscal rim thereby adding to the severity of the original lesion and special care should be taken not to cut too deeply into the meniscus when the rim is trimmed. Although the remaining rim may look irregular, particularly in the posterior third, attempts to trim it to perfection are likely to damage the articular cartilage (Fig. 8.2) and the surgeon should content himself with removing the offending fragment of meniscus and leaving a healthy rim rather than trying to paint the lily by removing insignificant fragments from the posterior horn and damaging the articular cartilage in the process.

The powered shaver can be used to 'contour' the irregularities of the rim and to remove debris (Fig. 6.50), but the shaver is not designed for this purpose and in the author's experience it is less effective than basket forceps or rongeurs. The powered meniscus cutter can also be used, but is unnecessarily vicious and its use could well result in the removal of more rim than necessary.

C. LATERAL MENISCUS

From the arthroscopic standpoint the anatomy of the lateral compartment differs from that of the medial in

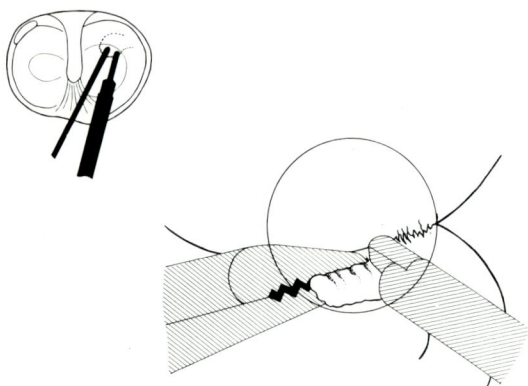

Fig. 6.43 An inferior flap of medial meniscus is grasped with forceps inserted from the antero-lateral route and divided at its base with the scissors of the operating arthroscope

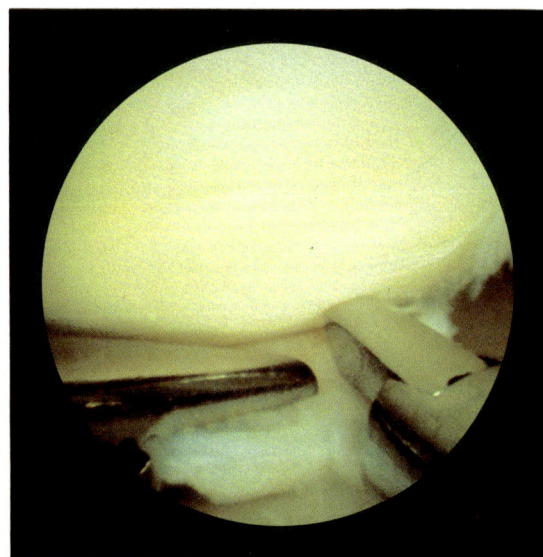

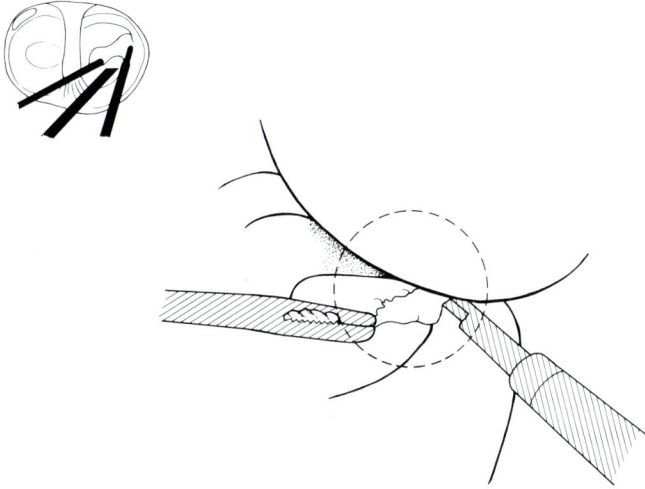

Fig. 6.44 Dividing the base of a long flap of medial meniscus using the triple puncture technique

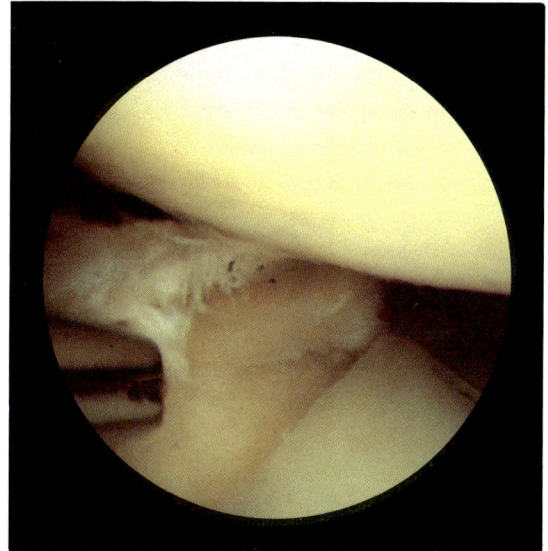

three important respects. Firstly, the anterior edge of the lateral tibial plateau lies a little lower than the medial and the lateral tibial plateau is domed so that its centre is higher than its periphery, while the reverse is true of the medial plateau. In consequence, instruments inserted immediately above the anterior horn of the lateral meniscus cannot be brought to bear upon the posterior horn, while those inserted from the antero-medial approach will easily do so if they are placed approximately 1 cm above the anterior edge

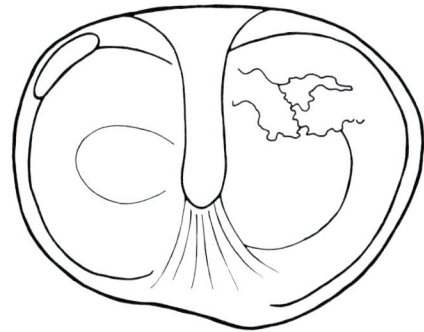

Fig. 6.45 Degenerate posterior horn of medial meniscus

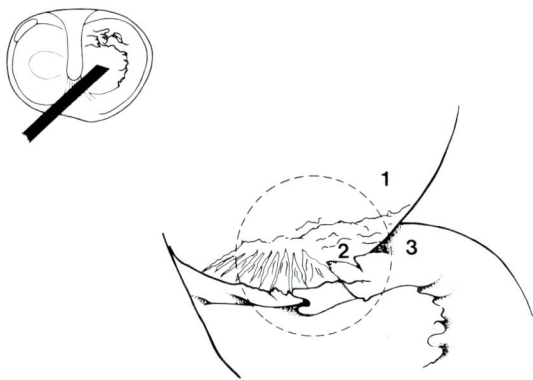

Fig. 6.46 A degenerate tear of the posterior horn of the medial meniscus (3) lying beneath an area of degenerate articular cartilage (2) on the under-surface of the medial femoral condyle (1)

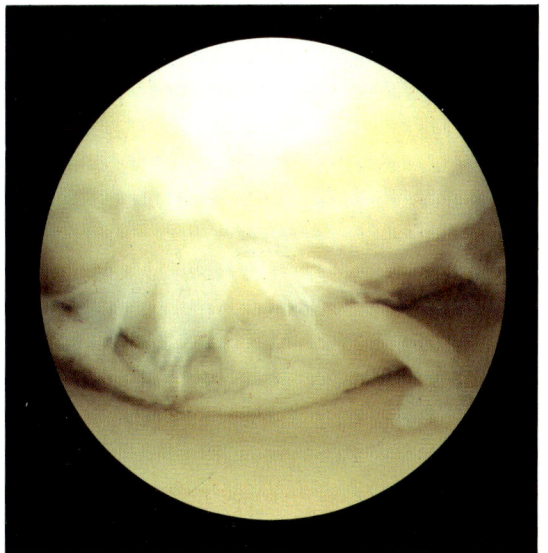

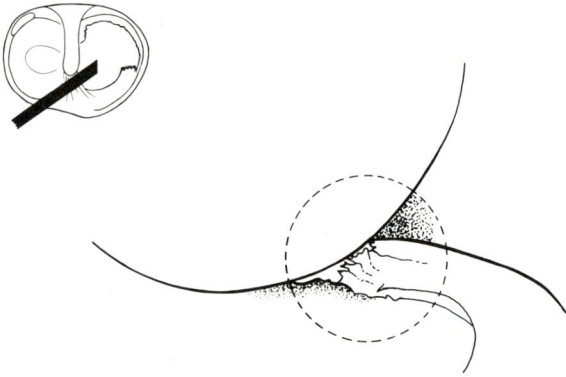

Fig. 6.47 The stump left after division of the anterior attachment of a bucket handle fragment of medial meniscus involving almost the whole width of the medial meniscus

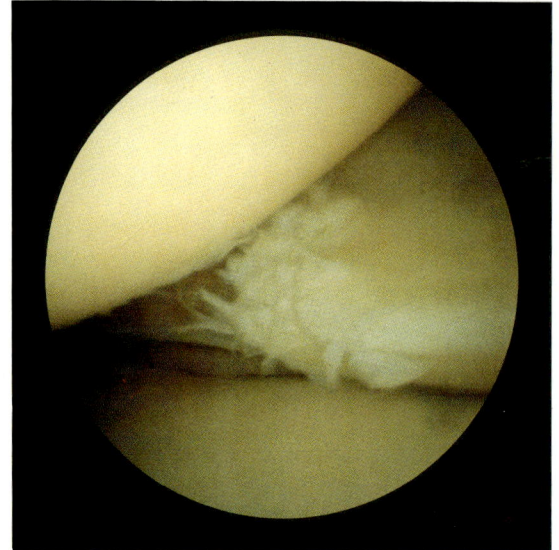

of the meniscus and close to the patellar tendon. Secondly, the lateral joint space can be opened more easily than can the lateral, and the tibial plateau itself is smaller so that access to the posterior part of the meniscus is relatively simple. Finally, the tunnel of the popliteus tendon acts as a localised 'peripheral separation' of the meniscus and influences the pattern of tears and the shape of the meniscal fragments.

The pattern of meniscal lesions in the lateral compartment also differs from that in the medial with a predominance of complex and oblique flaps involving both surfaces of the meniscus. Cystic degeneration is more common in the lateral meniscus than the medial, and discoid menisci are for practical purposes a lesion of the lateral meniscus only. Because of these differences in the anatomy and pathology of the lateral and medial compartments, lesions in the lateral compartment cannot be approached in the same way as those in the medial compartment.

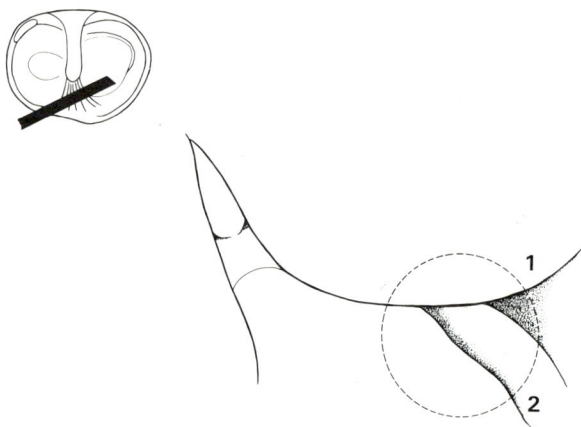

Fig. 6.48 The appearance of a medial meniscus (2) 12 months after removal of an incomplete (Type 2) tear of the medial meniscus. The step in the meniscus has become smooth, but the posterior part of the meniscus is narrower than the anterior part—(1) medial femoral condyle

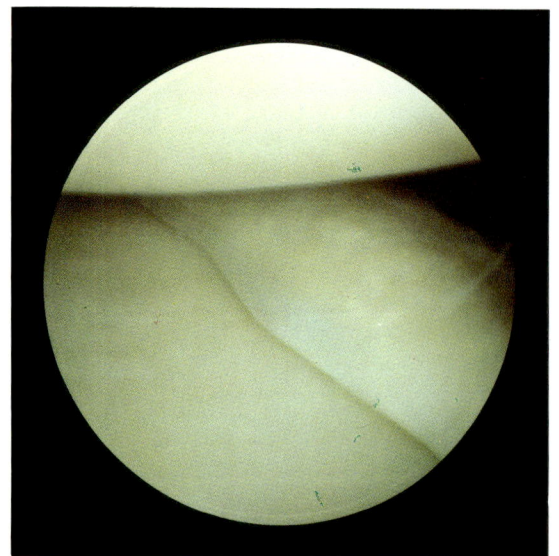

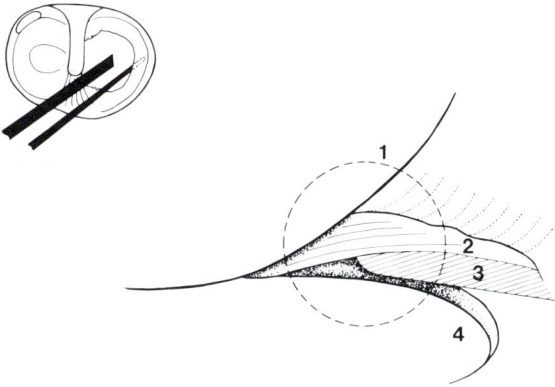

Fig. 6.49 Checking the integrity of the remaining meniscal rim (2) using a blunt hook (3)—(1) medial femoral condyle (4) medial tibial plateau

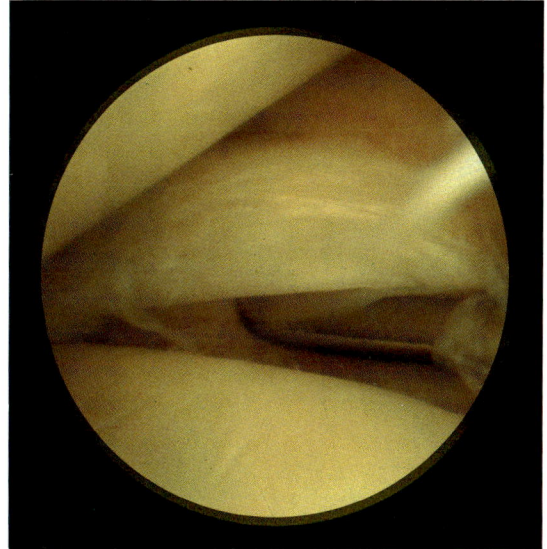

Circumferential tears

Identifying the anatomy

The circumferential vertical tear. An important difference between medial and lateral circumferential tears is the length of the fragment. The inner margin of the lateral meniscus is shorter than the medial with the result that bucket handle fragments are also shorter and the yield of meniscal tissue from the excision of a bucket handle fragment correspond-ingly smaller. Moreover, circumferential tears, which are less common in the lateral compartment than in the medial, follow a slightly different pattern. Although the tear almost always extends up to the posterior meniscal attachment or close to it, the anterior extent of the tear tends to be either at the anterior edge of the popliteus tunnel (Figs. 6.53, 6.54) or at the anterior attachment of the meniscus (Figs. 6.51. 6.52) and not at points in between, making it easy to determine the anterior extent of the tear.

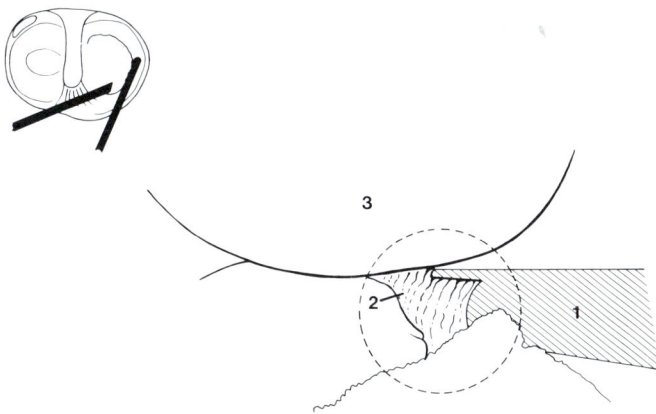

Fig. 6.50 Trimming an irregular meniscal rim (2) using the Stryker shaver (1)—(3) medial femoral condyle

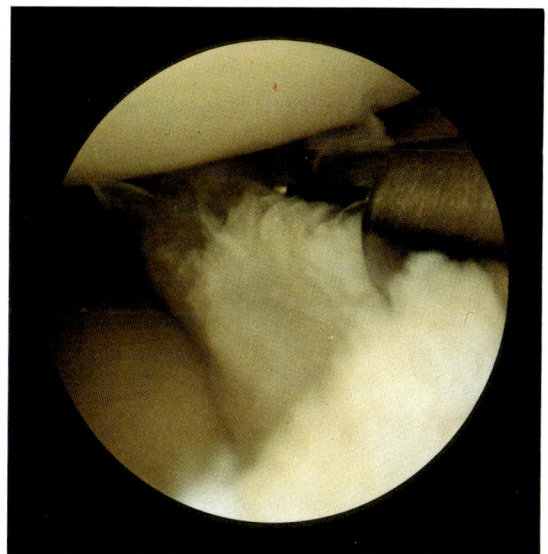

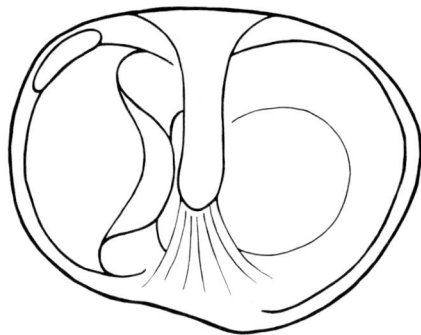

Fig. 6.51 A displaced bucket handle tear of the lateral meniscus involving its entire width and whole length

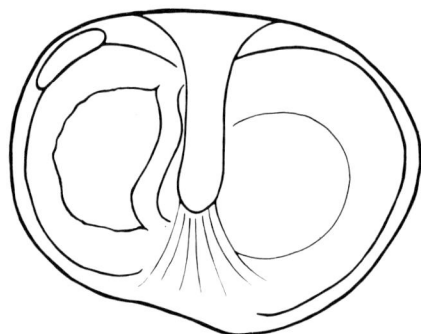

Fig. 6.53 A bucket handle tear involving the whole thickness of the lateral meniscus in its posterior half

The fragment itself may include the whole width of the meniscus (Figs. 6.51, 6.53) or only part of it (Figs. 6.52, 6.54). Fragments which involve the whole width of the meniscus usually affect the posterior half of the meniscus only, and acute tears of this type can be associated with haemarthrosis caused by bleeding from a small synovial tear at the anterior edge of the popliteus tunnel. This does not occur in tears that involve the body of the meniscus only.

Posterior third tears of the medial meniscus cause an abnormal prominence of the posterior edge of the meniscus when a valgus and external rotation force is applied. No such prominence occurs with similar tears of the lateral meniscus, but a percutaneous needle passed into the meniscus behind the popliteus tendon or a blunt hook passed under the meniscus will demonstrate tears in this area most effectively. The mobility of the lateral meniscus varies from person to person and can be difficult to assess, but a meniscus that remains dislocated in front of the condyle when the hook is removed must be considered pathological.

The circumferential horizontal tear. Horizontal tears extending from the free edge of the meniscus

to its periphery can produce a 'bucket handle' fragment including only the upper (Fig. 6.55), or more rarely, the lower half of the meniscus. Tears of this pattern are rare in the medial compartment, but are not uncommon in the lateral. Arthroscopically the only evidence of the tear may be a horizontal fissure on the free edge of the meniscus and a hook or needle is usually needed to demonstrate the exact anatomy of the tear.

Ruptured bucket handle tears. Unlike bucket handle fragments of the medial meniscus which usually become detached at or near the posterior attachment, those in the lateral compartment often break in their centre (Fig. 6.56) to produce various patterns of flap. Fragments which have become detached anteriorly can come to lie in the postero-lateral compartment and their presence should be suspected if the lateral meniscus is unusually narrow without any corresponding fragment. Tags arising from rupture of the fragment at its centre will usually have a characteristic square end (Fig. 6.57). It is important to recognise this appearance because such tags almost always occur in pairs, one arising from the

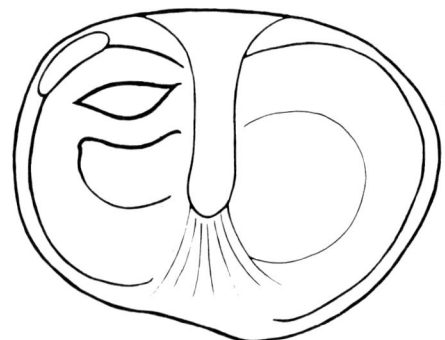

Fig. 6.52 A displaced bucket handle tear of the lateral meniscus involving part of its width and extending the whole length of the meniscus

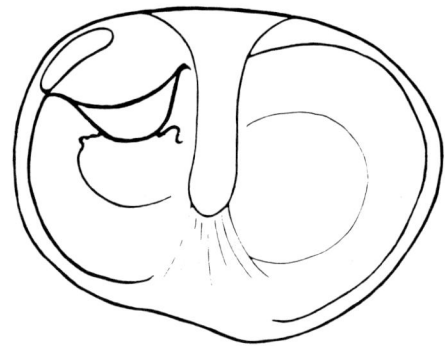

Fig. 6.54 A bucket handle tear involving part of the thickness of the posterior half of the lateral meniscus only

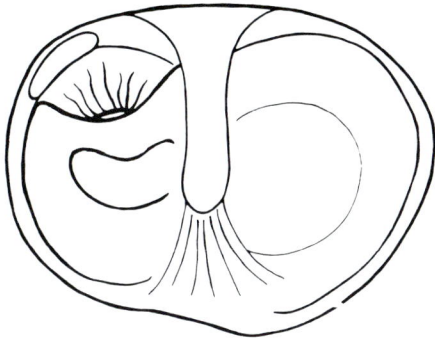

Fig. 6.55 A fragment of the upper surface of the lateral meniscus arising from a horizontal circumferential tear, leaving the inferior surface of the meniscus intact

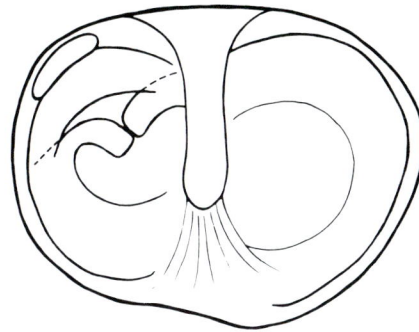

Fig. 6.56 A bucket handle fragment of the lateral meniscus ruptured in its centre

posterior end of the fragment and one from the anterior; both must be removed.

Removing the fragments

Fragments involving the whole length of the meniscus. As with bucket handle fragments in the medial compartment, the fragment should be divided at each end and removed. The procedure can be more difficult in the lateral compartment because it is smaller and tighter than the medial compartment so that a bucket handle fragment firmly locked in front of the condyle will occupy most of the available joint space (Fig. 6.58) and obstruct movement of the instruments, but the techniques outlined for the medial meniscus are nevertheless applicable to the lateral. Either the triple puncture technique or the

operating arthroscope can also be used, but it is the author's preference to use the simple double puncture technique.

Narrow fragments involving only part of the meniscal width and lying in the intercondylar notch can be removed in the same way as complete (Type I) tears of the medial meniscus by dividing the posterior horn with scissors and then avulsing the anterior attachment with rongeurs. Instruments inserted from the antero-medial approach close to the patellar tendon and above the meniscus will reach most parts of the lateral compartment, but the instruments and arthroscope usually need to be transposed when the posterior attachment is divided. Full-width fragments lying in the notch can also be removed in this way, but may be so tough and thick that they need to be divided

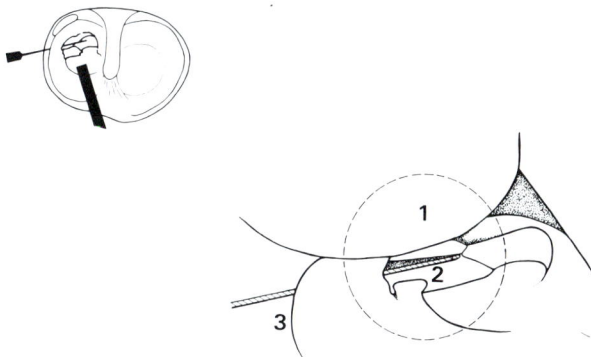

Fig. 6.57 A bucket handle fragment of the lateral meniscus ruptured at its centre (2) lying beneath the lateral femoral condyle (1) and probed with a percutaneous needle (3)

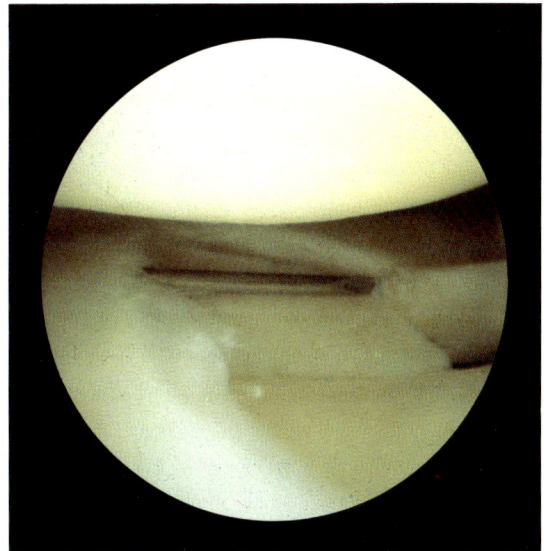

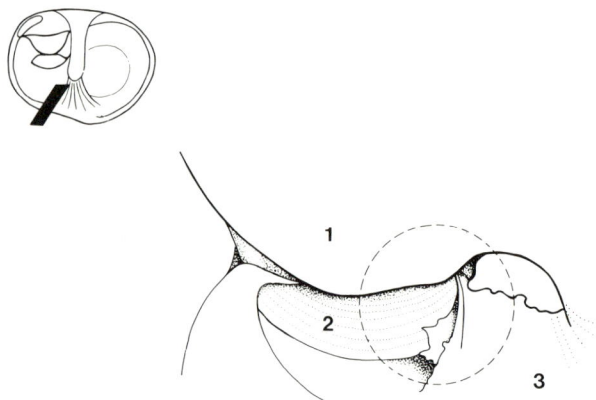

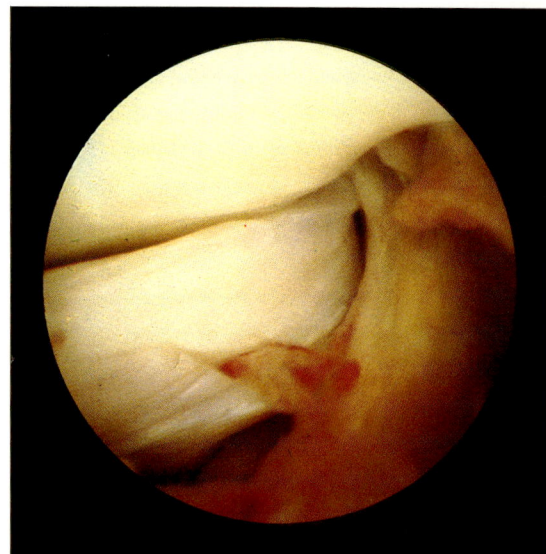

Fig. 6.58 The full thickness of the posterior half of the lateral meniscus (2) has come forward to lie beneath the lateral femoral condyle (1)—(3) anterior cruciate ligament

anteriorly with the scissors, knife, or guillotine, and the rest of the meniscus removed piecemeal with rongeurs.

Fragments involving posterior part of meniscus only. Tears that extend only to the anterior limit of the popliteus tunnel produce fragments that can become so tightly locked in front of the condyle that it is impossible to slip instruments between the condyle and fragment without damaging the articular cartilage (Fig. 8.2). These fragments can be divided at their anterior end with a guillotine passed under the fragment into the axilla of the tear, or with curved pituitary rongeurs passed above the fragment with the beak turned downwards to nibble through the fragment from its upper surface.

When the fragment has finally been divided anteriorly, a long posteriorly based stub will be left which can be removed with rongeurs applied at its base, but the fragment will tend to slip back into its normal position under the femoral condyle from which it must be retrieved with a hook. The fragment may also slip back through the notch into the postero-lateral compartment where it can be difficult to detect its presence, or into the recess beneath the posterior horn of the meniscus. If a large fragment appears to dematerialise in this way, the surgeon may be tempted to think that the fragment he believed he had seen earlier was some kind of mirage. Such a temptation must be resisted and the search continued with needle

hook and probe until the fragment is found (Fig. 6.59).

Although removal of the loose fragment is the standard treatment for such lesions at present, reattachment may well prove to be preferable. Even if the meniscus eventually becomes detached again and needs to be removed after a few years, the articular cartilage will at least have been protected for a few more years of the patient's active life.

Horizontal circumferential tears. Partial thickness bucket handle fragments arising from horizontal tears can be removed in the same way as those involving the whole thickness of the meniscus, but the initial division of the fragment is more difficult and can be done most easily with a guillotine or, if this is not available, with a knife blade slipped under the fragment. As in the medial compartment, it is important not to divide the rim completely and produce an unstable rim.

Ruptured bucket handle fragments. As in the medial compartment, fragments arising from ruptured bucket handle tears can be removed with rongeurs, punch forceps, or with the scissors of the operating arthroscope while the fragment is held with grasping forceps inserted from the antero-medial approach. It is the author's preference to use rongeurs (Fig. 6.60) or punch forceps rather than fiddle with the tunnel vision and feeble instruments of the operating arthroscope.

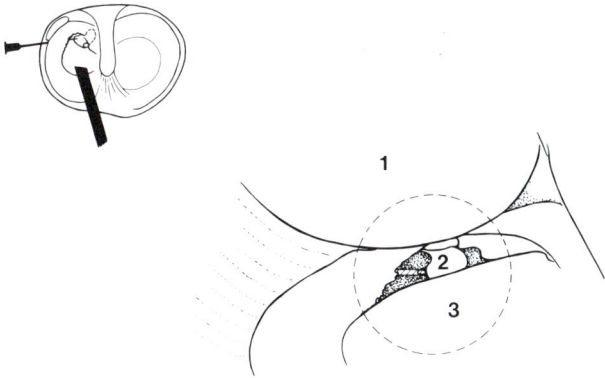

Fig. 6.59 A flap tear of lateral meniscus (2) has slipped backwards beneath the lateral femoral condyle (1) and behind the lateral tibial plateau (3), and is manipulated with a percutaneous needle

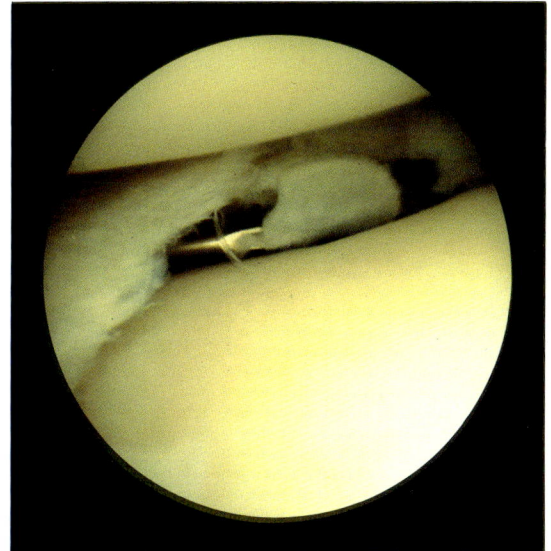

Checking the rim

Just as with the medial meniscus, the stability of the rim must be checked carefully after the fragment has been removed, but in the lateral compartment special attention must be paid to the popliteus tunnel. If the fragment involves the whole thickness of the meniscus, the popliteus tendon will be exposed without any bridge of tissue crossing it so that the rim of the meniscus is completely divided and functionless. In

these circumstances, any remaining meniscal tissue is redundant and is not only useless but likely to become degenerate, swollen and painful, causing a block to extension which will not be relieved until the remaining tissue is removed. Accordingly, as much meniscal tissue as possible should be removed if the popliteus tendon is completely exposed throughout its passage through the knee.

If there is a good bridge of intact tissue across the tendon (Fig. 6.61) trimming of the rim in this area

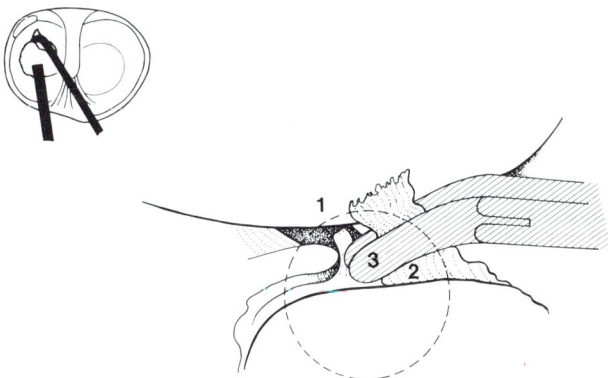

Fig. 6.60 Trimming the fragments of a torn lateral meniscus (2) using curved pituitary rongeurs opposite the popliteus tunnel—(1) lateral femoral condyle

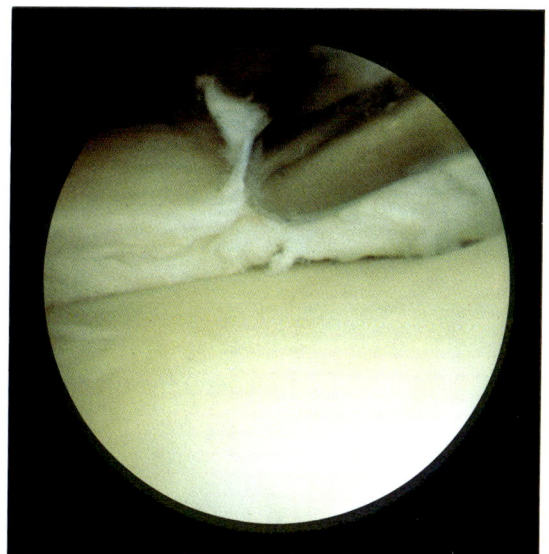

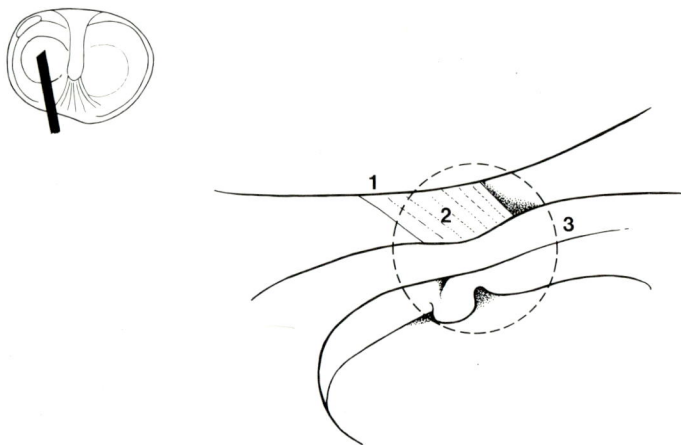

Fig. 6.61 A good bridge of lateral meniscus (3) crossing the popliteus tendon (2). Note the horizontal fissure in the centre of the lateral meniscus—(1) lateral femoral condyle

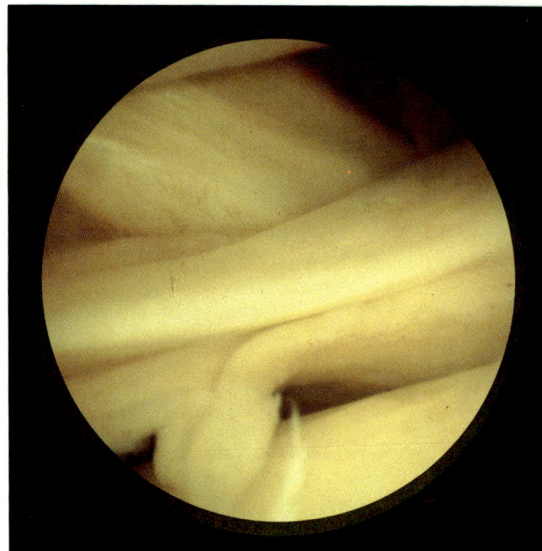

must be kept to an absolute minimum because it is only too easy for the bridge to be divided completely in the course of over-enthusiastic trimming, and even for the popliteus tendon itself to be damaged (Fig. 6.62). Irregularities of the rim in front of the popliteus tunnel and behind it can be trimmed firmly back to healthy tissue without worry, but even a slender popliteus bridge is worth preserving and it is probably better to leave the popliteus bridge a little rough rather than risk dividing it completely.

Flaps and tags

Identifying the anatomy

Flaps and tags in the lateral compartment differ radically from those found in the medial compartment, with a rich profusion of oblique tears influenced by the presence of the popliteus tunnel.

Anterior tags. Anteriorly based tags can arise from a vertical split in the meniscus that runs backwards for a variable distance to the free margin

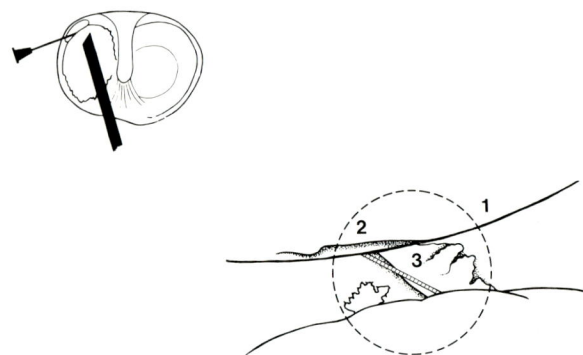

Fig. 6.62 Over-enthusiastic trimming of the lateral meniscal rim has damaged the popliteus tendon (3). Longstanding degenerative change (2) is visible on the under-surface of the lateral femoral condyle (1)

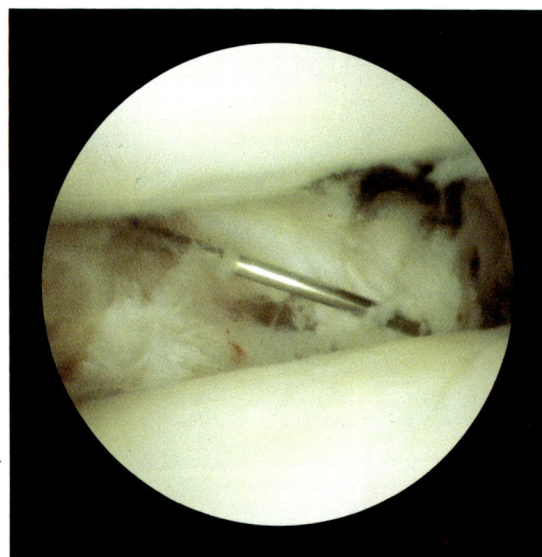

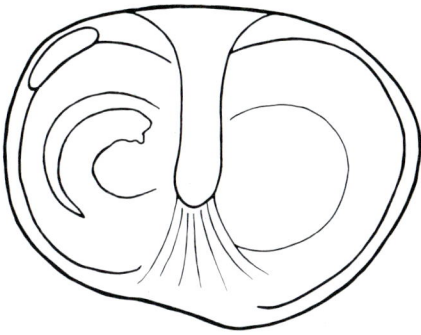

Fig. 6.63 An anterior horn tag of the lateral meniscus

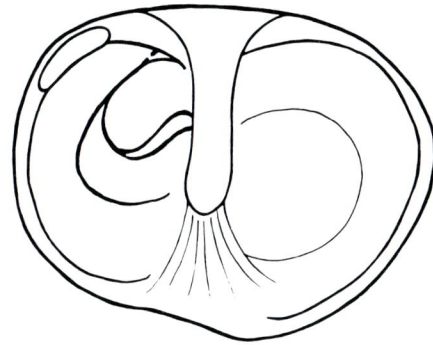

Fig. 6.64 A large flap of the posterior third of the lateral meniscus involving the full meniscal thickness

of the meniscus, creating a flap that can cause locking and clicking out of all proportion to its size (Fig. 6.63).

Exact definition of the anatomy of these lesions can be difficult because the fragment lies so close to the lens that it may be confused with a bucket handle tear, or even with a mass of distended synovium. The exact anatomy can be established by passing the arthroscope beyond the fragment of tissue at the front of the joint into the back of the lateral compartment, and examining the free margin of the meniscus. Loss of the clean, sharp meniscal edge may be seen in the anterior part of the joint and closer inspection will demonstrate that the tissue at the front of the joint corresponds with the defect in the meniscus, and is in fact, an anterior meniscal tag.

Posterior flaps. Horizontal or slightly oblique splits in the posterior part of the meniscus can separate a large chunk of tissue from the posterior horn (Figs. 6.64, 6.65) which may be so thick that the flap itself is thicker than the remaining rim. Flaps of this pattern are attached posteriorly, and can be manipulated easily with a percutaneous needle or hook.

Oblique flap tears and parrot beaks. Most meniscal flaps in the lateral compartment result from tears that run obliquely through the meniscal substance from above posteriorly to below anteriorly. The resulting split appears as a curved radial tear on the upper surface of the meniscus (Fig. 6.66) and an oblique tear on the free margin so that when the meniscus is excised at open operation the two sections of meniscus slide over each other to produce the classical 'parrot-beak' appearance (Figs. 6.67 (a) & (b), 6.68).

The behaviour of the flap is dictated by the position

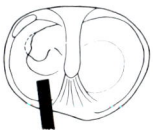

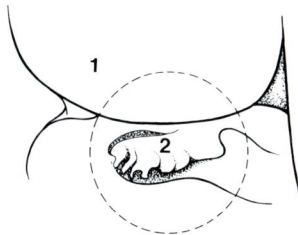

Fig. 6.65 A large flap of lateral meniscus (2) has come forward to lie beneath the lateral femoral condyle as the result of a 'parrot-beak tear' entering the popliteus tunnel

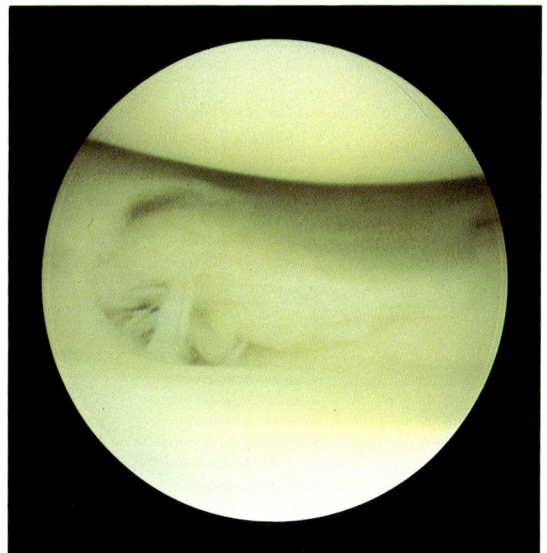

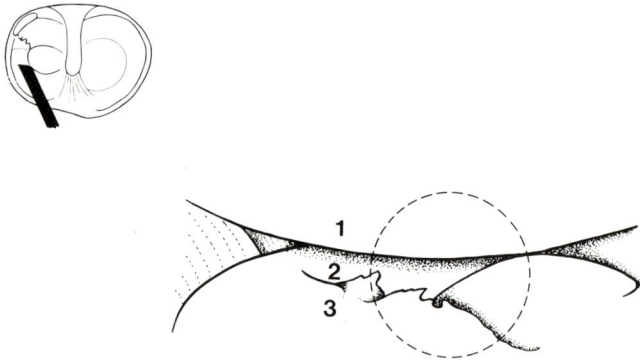

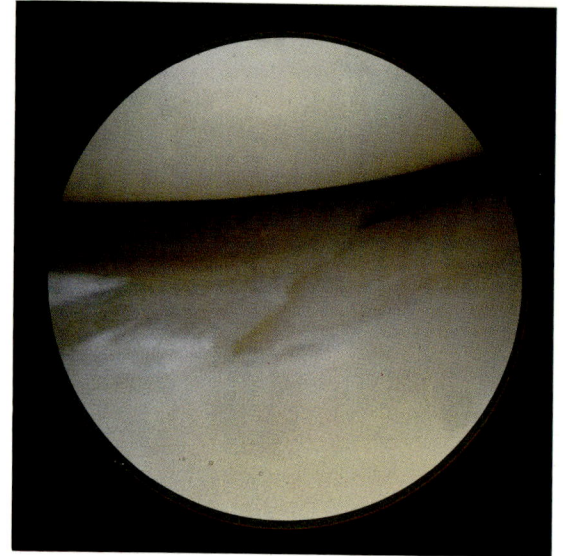

Fig. 6.66 A tear (2) in the lateral meniscus (3) lying anterior to the popliteus tunnel is tethered so that it cannot move into the joint space—(1) lateral femoral condyle

of the tear and its relationship to the popliteus tunnel. If the lower and anterior end of the tear lies opposite the popliteus tunnel, the flap will be free to move in and out of the joint (Fig. 6.69) or become tucked back on itself to lie under the popliteus tendon, where it will be found as a fusiform swelling on the lateral joint line and may be wrongly diagnosed as a cyst of the meniscus. If the split on the lower surface of the meniscus lies in front of the popliteus tunnel, the flap will be tethered to the lateral side of the knee at its anterior edge (Fig. 6.70) and will not be able to move into the centre of the joint.

Very occasionally, the split on the upper surface of the meniscus also lies in front of the popliteus tunnel without extending through to the lower surface, producing a thin sliver of meniscus raised from the upper surface of the meniscus (Fig. 6.71).

Apart from the relationship of the flap to the popliteus tunnel, these tears also vary according to their lateral extent, some tears extending right

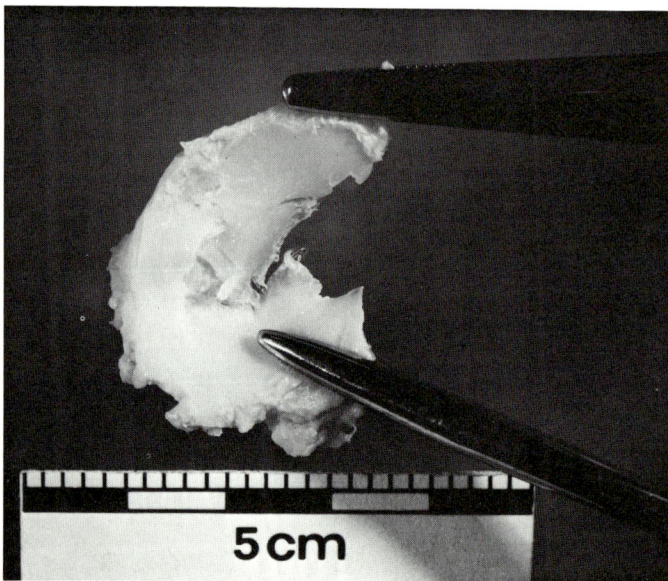

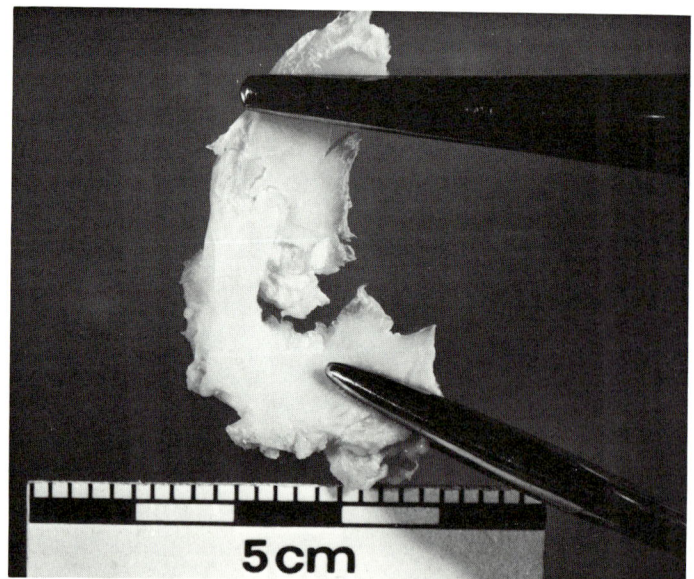

Fig. 6.67 (a) 'parrot-beak' tear of the lateral meniscus held in the anatomical position, (b) the meniscus opened to demonstrate the plane of cleavage extending into the popliteus tunnel

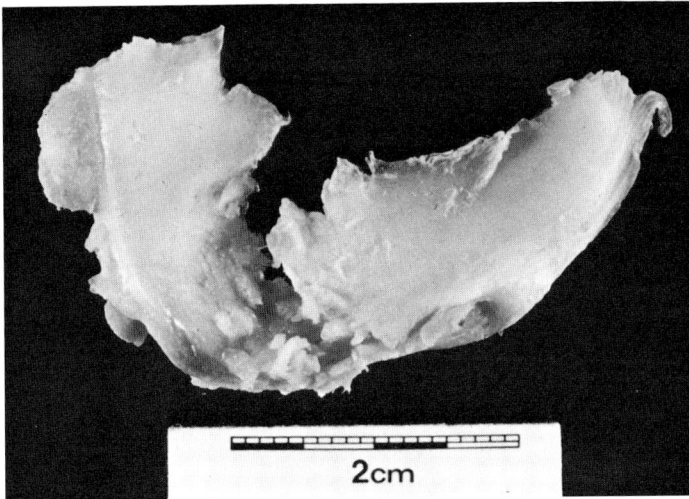

Fig. 6.68 The inferior surface of the meniscus shown in Figure 6.67, demonstrating the complete rupture of the meniscal rim on the inferior surface

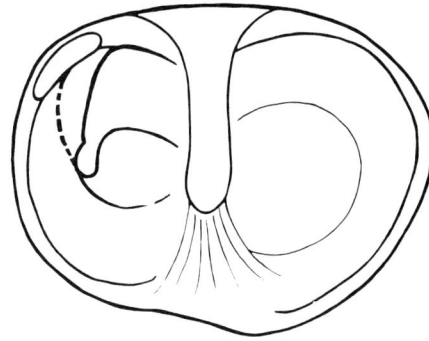

Fig. 6.69 A 'parrot-beak' tear entering the popliteus tunnel, allowing the lower fragment to move into the joint space

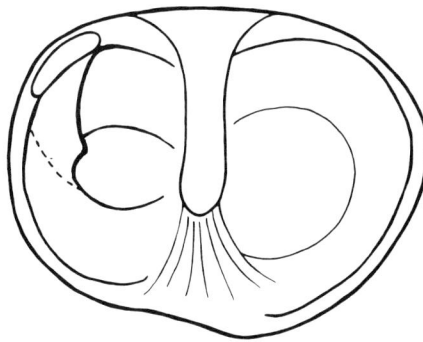

Fig. 6.70 A 'parrot-beak' tear lying in front of the popliteus tunnel tethering the inferior fragment so that it is not free to move into the joint space

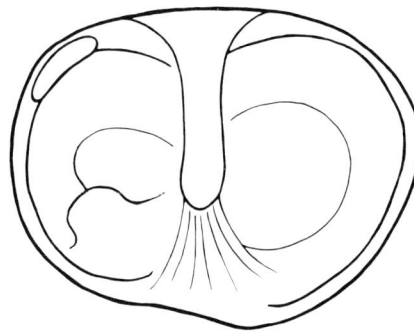

Fig. 6.71 An inferior oblique tear of the lateral meniscus involving the upper surface only

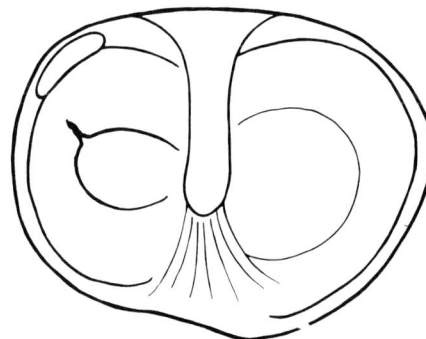

Fig. 6.72 A small radial split of the lateral meniscus

through the rim and some only part of the way. It is important to discover the depth, or lateral extent, of the tear before operating instruments are inserted.

Radial tears. Small radial splits on the free margin of the lateral meniscus and in its mid-portion are sometimes seen, and are hard to relate to the patient's symptoms (Fig. 6.72). These lesions perhaps represent the beginnings of a parrot-beak tear.

The 'shattered' lateral meniscus. Apart from the isolated flaps, splits and tears described above, multiple splits and flaps also occur and leave a tattered fringe of torn meniscal tissue for which the only solution is total meniscectomy. When such a meniscus is found, it can either be removed *secundum artem* with grasping forceps, punch forceps and rongeurs, or according to the technique of total meniscectomy described earlier. Special care must be taken not to damage the articular cartilage while removing the last crumbs of degenerate tissue.

Removing the fragment and checking the rim

Tears extending completely through the meniscus into the popliteus tunnel on both upper and lower surfaces sever the rim of the meniscus completely, leaving no alternative to trimming back as much of the meniscus as possible both anteriorly and posteriorly with punch forceps and rongeurs, but if the tear extends only part of the way through the rim, the meniscus can be trimmed back cautiously until the base of the tear is exposed and a gently curving rim is

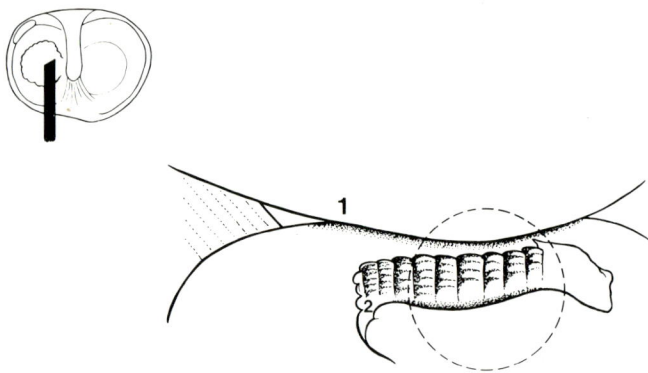

Fig. 6.73 The trimmed rim of a lateral meniscal tear (2) involving part of the meniscal thickness only—(1) lateral femoral condyle

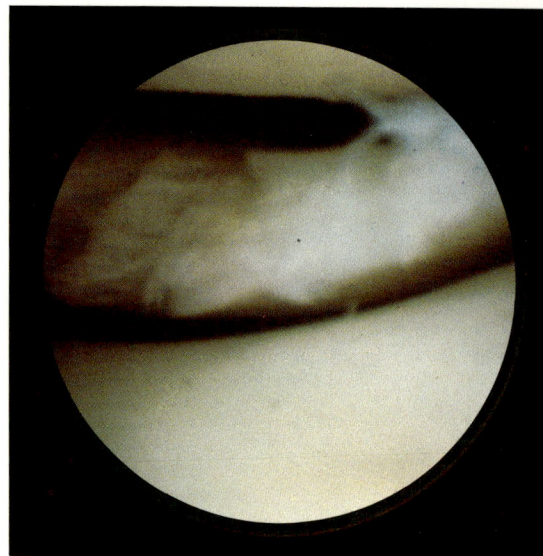

achieved (Fig. 6.73). As with circumferential tears, it is easy to enter the popliteus tunnel and divide the rim completely by misplaced enthusiasm in the trimming of the rim.

Tears in the posterior part of the meniscus which result in a free flap should be dealt with by removing the flap as a first step and then assessing the rim. If it is found that a bridge of healthy tissue is left crossing the popliteus tunnel, the edges of the bridge can be trimmed lightly, preserving as much of the peripheral rim as possible, but if no such bridge is present the remaining meniscal tissue should also be removed.

Partial thickness flaps split from the upper surface of the meniscus in its anterior third are best treated by gentle trimming with fine punch forceps or scissors. An alternative is to grasp the free edge of the flap with curved pituitary rongeurs and peel the flap back to the anterior meniscal attachment from which it can be removed more neatly.

Other lesions of the lateral meniscus

Radial tears

Although there is no evidence that small radial tears are the source of symptoms or that cutting them back to their base prevents major tears developing, the procedure is simple and unlikely to cause harm. The tear should be cut with basket forceps or punch forceps until its base is reached, and no further. The edge of the defect should then be trimmed to leave a gently curving meniscal margin, taking care that no more tissue is removed than absolutely necessary.

Discoid menisci

An intact discoid meniscus may give rise to nothing more remarkable than asymptomatic loss of extension, but lateral meniscectomy may well be followed by osteoarthrosis. Because the knee with an intact discoid meniscus has a better future than a knee with no lateral meniscus at all, a discoid meniscus should not be excised unless it is the source of symptoms bad enough to warrant operation.

Symptoms can be caused by at least two types of lesions in discoid menisci. In the first, the upper surface of the meniscus becomes torn with the development of irregular flaps (Fig. 6.74 (a) & (b)) and clefts that do not penetrate to the lower surface of the meniscus and in the second, a split develops in the centre of the meniscus to create a fragment which is effectively an enormous locked bucket handle fragment (Figs. 6.75, 6. 76).

Tears of both types can be treated arthroscopically by excision of the central portion of the meniscus to leave an intact rim. The excision of fragments involving the whole thickness of the meniscus is most easily done with punch forceps starting in the intercondylar notch and working laterally, but division of the anterior attachment starting in the central defect is an alternative (Fig. 6.77). The aim of excision

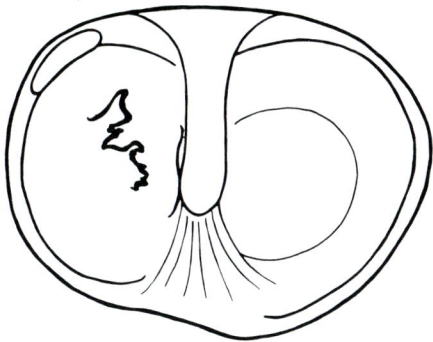

Fig. 6.74 A tear of a lateral discoid meniscus involving the upper surface only, and (b) a specimen obtained by open meniscectomy

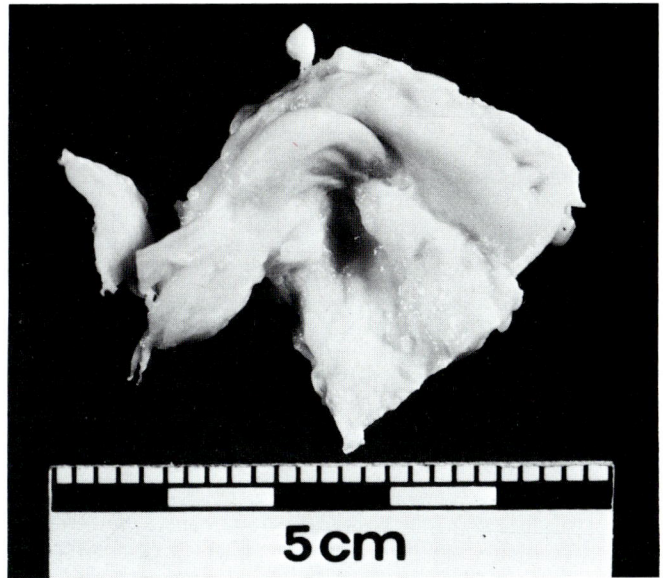

should be, as always, an intact and stable rim, but with the difference that the resulting rim will be of the same width as a normal meniscus rather than narrower (Fig. 6.78). The operation is not difficult provided that it is done carefully and methodically.

If arthroscopy reveals irregularity of the upper surface of the meniscus only, the damaged tissue in the central portion of the meniscus can be removed piecemeal with punch forceps and rongeurs beginning at the free margin in the intercondylar notch and working laterally. This procedure is more difficult than excision of a completely torn discoid meniscus

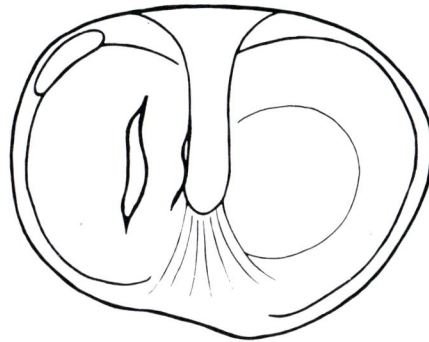

Fig. 6.75 A discoid lateral meniscus with a tear involving its full thickness

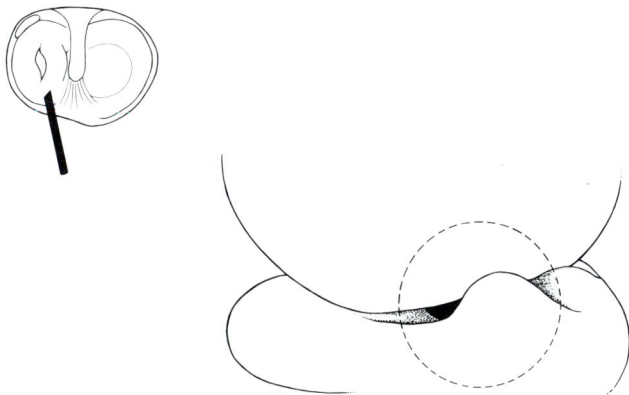

Fig. 6.76 A tear involving the full thickness of a discoid lateral meniscus, with the mobile fragment lying in the intercondylar notch and seen from the antero-lateral approach

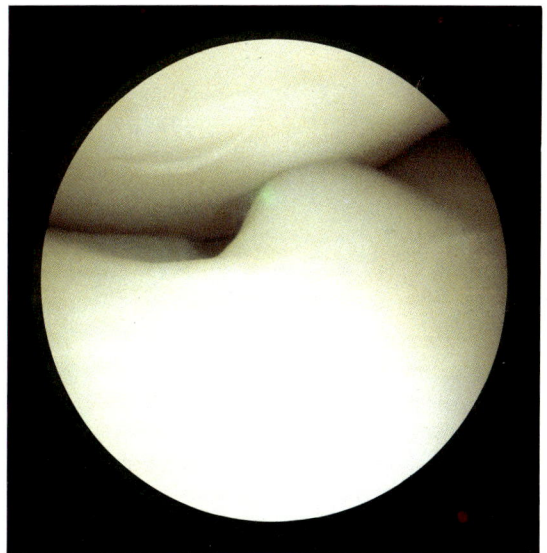

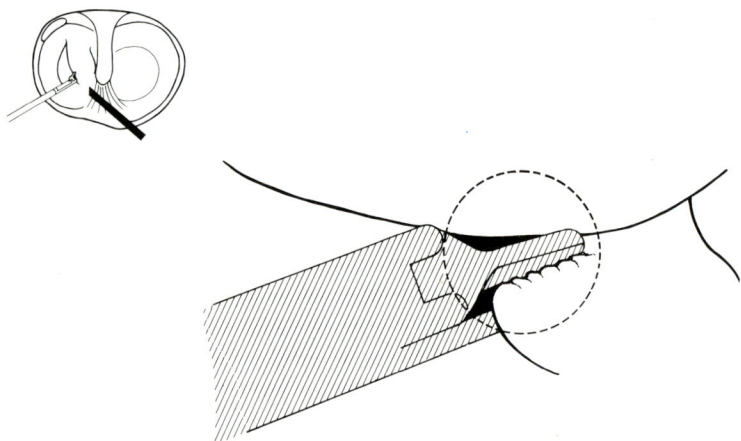

Fig. 6.77 Cutting the anterior attachment of the fragment shown in Figure 6.76, using scissors inserted from the antero-lateral approach, and with the arthroscope inserted from the antero-medial approach

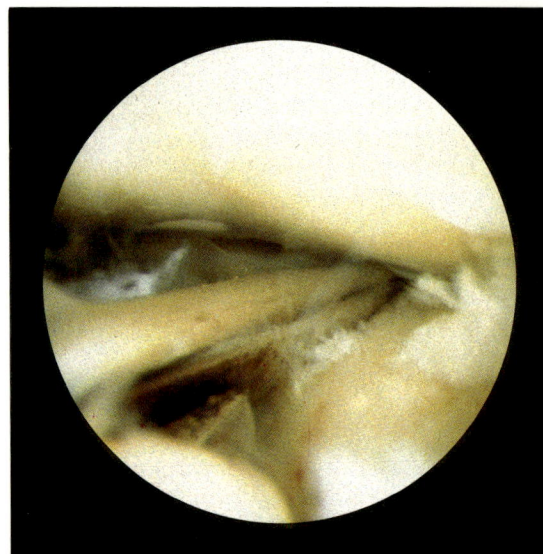

and results in many small fragments of meniscal tissue in the joint, all of which must be removed. An alternative is to excise the centre of the meniscus with the scissors of the operating arthroscope while traction is applied with forceps inserted from the antero-medial approach, but the bulk of the meniscus makes this difficult.

Cystic degeneration

If the patient is troubled by pain, tenderness and swelling along the lateral jointline rather than by the mechanical symptoms of a meniscal tear, cystic degeneration of the meniscus must be suspected (Fig. 6.79).

The arthroscopic appearance of a meniscus affected by cystic degeneration is often unremarkable. A few small fissures may be noted on the upper surface or free margin of the meniscus and the usually smooth knife-like edge may be blunted so that the meniscus presents a swollen and somewhat bloated appearance (Fig. 6.80). Although the arthroscopic appearance

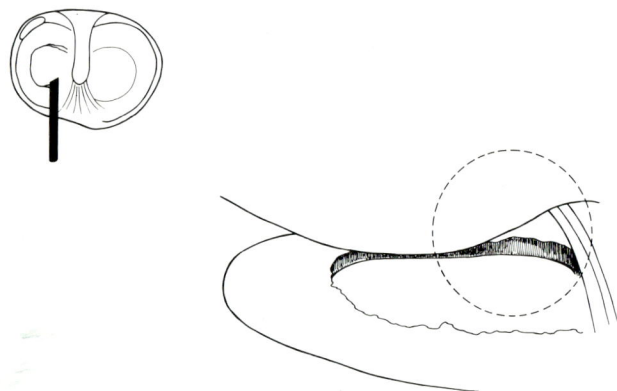

Fig. 6.78 The rim of the meniscus shown in Figure 6.76 after removal of the mobile fragment

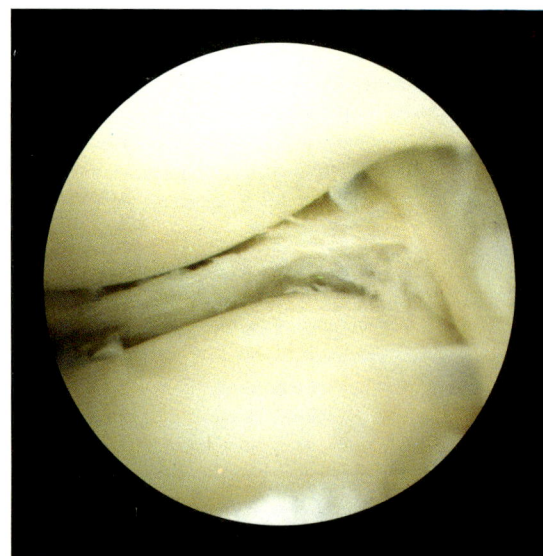

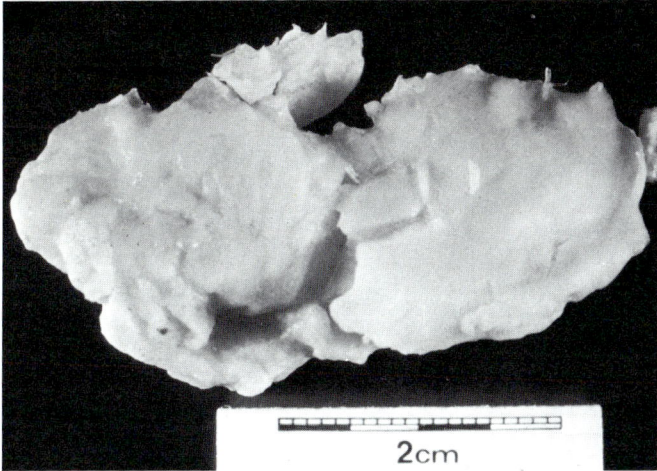

Fig. 6.79 A lateral meniscus affected by cystic degeneration (removed by open meniscectomy)

may be unhelpful, the clinical features of pain, jointline tenderness and swelling should have alerted the surgeon to the possible diagnosis long before the patient reached the operating theatre.

Total removal of a cystic meniscus is more difficult than excision of a discoid meniscus because cystic menisci do not split along the grain of their fibres in the same way as healthy menisci with a single tear. The tissue has a rubbery and slightly 'springy' feel, and there is a very real possibility of fracturing the operating instruments by taking excessively large bites of tissue, or twisting the instruments. Unless the entire meniscus can be converted to a single large

bucket handle fragment, excision is simply a matter of patient persistence and painstaking piecemeal excision. Neither of these techniques is entirely satisfactory, and it is the author's opinion that the ideal arthroscopic technique for gross cystic degeneration of the lateral meniscus has yet to be found.

Solitary 'cysts' of the meniscus

The author must admit to being puzzled by the very considerable differences that exist between practical experience of meniscal cysts and the standard teaching on the subject. Although solitary cysts of the lateral meniscus undoubtedly do occur, in the author's experience the majority of isolated swellings 1 to 2 centimetres in diameter found on the lateral joint line and most obvious in slight flexion of the knee prove to be the result of a specific pattern of meniscal tear involving the inferior surface of the meniscus, and not a cyst. The fragments created by these tears are based anteriorly in such a way that they can be forced laterally to lie in front of the popliteus tendon, where they can be felt as a swelling on the lateral joint line (Fig. 6.81 (a)). Clinical examination of these swellings usually shows that they can be made to disappear by pushing the 'cyst' medially with the thumb while the knee is held in varus and that it will stay absent until a valgus and rotational strain is applied, when it will reappear. Arthroscopic examination shows synovitis and a characteristic bulge at the anterior edge of the

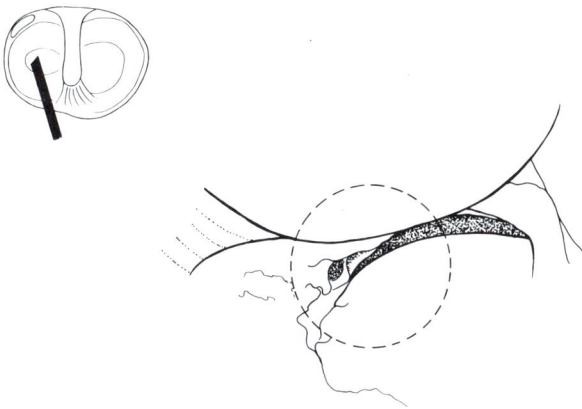

Fig. 6.80 Cystic degeneration of the lateral meniscus

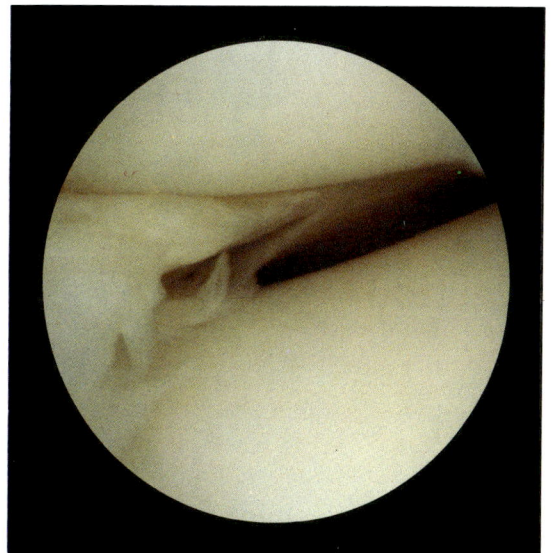

(a)   (b)

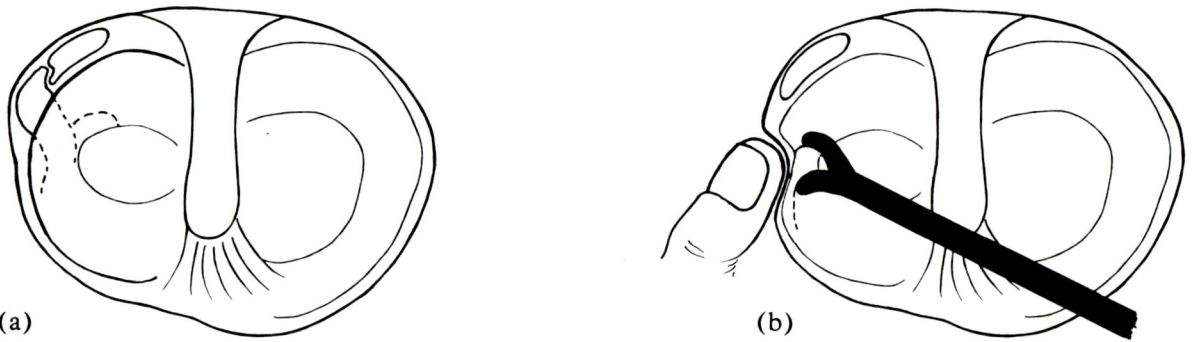

Fig. 6.81 (a) The position of an inferior flap of lateral meniscus mimicking a solitary cyst of the meniscus and (b) the position of the rongeurs for the removal of such a flap

popliteus tunnel. As further evidence for the suggestion that these 'cysts' are in fact meniscal tags of an unusual pattern, there are the observations that they are invariably associated with a tear on the inferior surface of the meniscus immediately in front of the popliteus tunnel, and that they can be removed with curved pituitary rongeurs inserted from the antero-medial approach and passed beneath the lateral meniscus. The lesion can be grasped, if necessary with the help of external finger pressure at the lateral joint line (Fig. 6.81 (b)) and avulsed to leave a meniscus that is intact on its upper surface, but with a defect on its inferior surface (Fig. 6.82). It is noticeable that both the joint line swelling and the patient's symptoms disappear immediately after such a procedure, but a long term study is needed to be sure that the lesions do not recur and that the meniscal rim remains intact.

If the joint line swelling does not disappear with a little thumb pressure and a varus strain and the meniscus is intact arthroscopically with a clear sharp edge, the swelling is probably a true cyst of the meniscus and must be excised through a short transverse incision splitting the iliotibial tract in the direction of its fibres, but not extending into the synovial cavity itself. Rehabilitation after such a limited excision is much simpler and swifter than after a formal arthrotomy, but slower than that which follows arthroscopic meniscectomy.

REFERENCES

Annandale T 1885 An operation for Displaced Semilunar Cartilage. British Medical Journal: 779.
Bonnin J G 1956 In Platt H (ed) Modern Trends in Orthopaedics, 2nd Series. Butterworth, London.

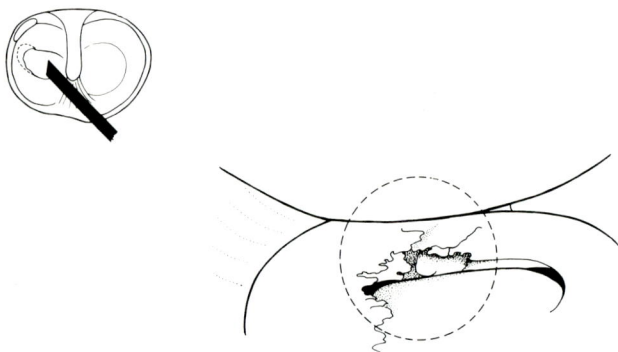

Fig. 6.82 The appearance of the lateral meniscus after excision of an inferior flap simulating a solitary cyst

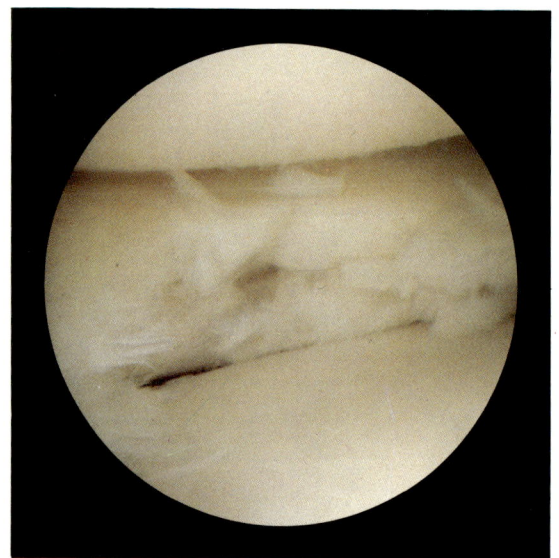

Bullough P, Munuera L, Murphy J, Weinstein A 1970 The strength of the menisci as it relates to their fine structure. Journal of Bone and Joint Surgery 52–B: 564–570.

Gear M 1967 The Late Results of Meniscectomy. British Journal of Surgery 54: 270–272.

Hargreaves D J, Seedhom B B 1979 On the 'bucket-handle' tear: Partial or total meniscectomy? A quantitative study. Journal of Bone and Joint Surgery 61–B: 381.

Huckell J 1965 Is Meniscectomy a Benign Procedure? A long-term follow-up study. Canadian Journal of Surgery 8: 254–260.

Jackson J P 1968 Degenerative changes in the knee after meniscectomy. British Medical Journal 2: 525–527.

Jones R 1909 Notes on derangements of the knee; based upon personal experience of over five hundred operations. Annals of Surgery 50: 969–1001.

Jones R E, Smith E C, Reisch J S 1978 Effects of Medial Meniscectomy on patients older than Forty Years. Journal of Bone and Joint Surgery 60A: 783–786.

McGinty J B, Geuss L F, Marvin R A 1977 Partial or Total Meniscectomy. A comparative analysis. Journal of Bone and Joint Surgery 59A: 763–766.

Oretorp N 1978 On the diagnosis and treatment of meniscus and ligament injuries in the knee. Linköping University Medical Dissertation No. 63, Linköping.

Seedhom B B, Wright V 1974 Functions of the menisci—A Preliminary Study 56–B: 381.

Smillie I S 1970 Injuries of the Knee Joint. 4th edn. Churchill Livingstone, Edinburgh.

Stone R G 1979 Peripheral Detachment of the Menisci of the Knee: A Preliminary Report. Orthopedic Clinics of North America 10: 643–657.

Tapper E, Hoover N 1969 Late results After Meniscectomy. Journal of Bone and Joint Surgery 51A: 517–526.

Zaman M, Leonard M A 1978 Meniscectomy in children: a study of fifty-nine knees. Journal of Bone and Joint Surgery 60–B: 436.

7

A system for learning arthroscopic surgery

Arthroscopic surgery requires considerable co-ordination of hand and eye and it has actually been suggested that some people are physically incapable of this kind of work. It is the author's opinion that this view is incorrect, and that apart from those unfortunate individuals who have one eye that is so incurably dominant that they are for practical purposes blind on one side, anybody who can perform standard orthopaedic procedures with reasonable competence is also capable of learning arthroscopic surgery. While different surgeons will progress at different rates and some will find the operations difficult and possibly uncongenial, the existence of a true physiological barrier that prevents some people from performing these procedures seems most improbable.

The learning of arthroscopic surgery, like the learning of arthroscopy itself, is a lonely business. Unless a dual viewing aid is available, the nature of the operation makes it impossible for anyone but the surgeon to observe the operation, with the inevitable result that arthroscopists are largely self-taught and learn only by repeating the mistakes of their predecessors. While there are many powerful arguments against such a haphazard system of learning, there is also the advantage that surgeons share the same experience as they learn and can therefore chart their progress with some accuracy. This fact is important because it is possible to relate the surgeon's experience to the operations that it is safe for him to attempt and allows the learning process to be conducted in a safe and orderly progression from the simplest operations to the most difficult.

Although the rate of learning will vary from one individual to the next, the following general outline of the successive stages of learning should be helpful as a guide to the order in which new techniques should be attempted, and when.

1. Arthroscopic honeymoon. The first five or ten arthroscopies are associated with the excitement and enthusiasm that come with the first experience of any new procedure. The underwater scenery of the knee can be spectacular and the beauty of the first clear glimpse down the arthroscope is a memorable moment that makes it easy to bear the inevitable early failures. This stage is short-lived.

2. Depression. In contrast to the previous period, the next 20 or 30 examinations are attended by gloom and disillusion. Early successes prove unrepeatable, the encroachment on available operating time becomes apparent, and the patience of the operating theatre staff begins to wear thin. No clinical benefit from the procedure can be seen, and there is a great temptation to abandon arthroscopy and return to the old ways that served so well before this new-fangled gadget came along. The decision to abandon arthroscopy is seldom made consciously at this stage but comes about more often by the gradual lengthening of the interval between arthroscopic attempts. The surgeon must recognise this temptation and overcome it if he is to succeed.

3. Success. Once the period of depression has passed—usually after some 40 or so attempts—the examination becomes more predictable and most of the knee will be seen in most of the patients. The findings of arthroscopy will generally be confirmed at arthrotomy and the surgeon will begin to have as much confidence in his arthroscopic technique as in his clinical judgement. During this period, anaesthetists and other colleagues will come to accept that arthroscopy is an inevitable time-wasting prelude to arthrotomy, and there is some justification for this belief because preliminary arthroscopy can do nothing but add to the theatre time required for a meniscectomy. Despite this criticism, the surgeon can at last expect to see some rewards for his efforts when the findings of arthroscopy allow him to make the incision for meniscectomy and other procedures more precisely.

The next great landmark comes when the decision is made not to proceed to arthrotomy, and to accept that the arthroscopic findings are more likely to be correct than the evidence of clinical and radiological investigations. When this step has been taken, usually after some 30 or 40 examinations, even the theatre staff will begin to see the real advantages of arthroscopy. Patients will be returned to the wards with their knees intact and knowledge of the exact pathology will allow the arthrotomies necessary in the rest of the patients to be done more swiftly and neatly than was previously possible.

4. Percutaneous needles. With the nursery slopes behind him, the surgeon can turn his attention to advanced diagnostic techniques as a prelude to arthroscopic surgery, and begin practising the techniques of holding the leg, and manipulating needles and instruments within the knee. It must be emphasised yet again that no attempt to excise a meniscus or to perform any other surgical procedure should be made until the surgeon is utterly confident in his arthroscopic findings and in the basic techniques of arthroscopic surgery.

The first and simplest 'exercise' is to identify the tip of the irrigation needle in the suprapatellar pouch. When the needle tip can be found easily and without conscious effort, it may be used to probe or manipulate structures in the supratellar pouch such as the medial suprapatellar plica, the undersurface of the patella, or the synovial shelf. Attempts to grasp and remove a loose body at this stage are unwise but it should be possible to transfix suitable loose bodies (Fig. 5.7) with a percutaneous needle so that they can be removed through a short arthrotomy. Orientation can be difficult at first and it may be helpful to revert to the straight-ahead 0° telescope rather than the 30° fore-oblique telescope.

The use of percutaneous probing needles along the joint-line should also be tried at this stage. The point of insertion is most easily found by looking at the desired point of entry through the arthroscope and placing the needle just below the point of trans-

illuminated skin as described in Chapter 2, but with the practice it becomes possible to place the needle in the correct position without taking the eye away from the eyepiece. The needle should be slipped either above or below the meniscus rather than into its substance, but insertion directly into the body of the meniscus itself may be needed to dislodge a concealed bucket handle fragment or to establish the presence of a lesion in the posterior horn. Gentle manipulation of the needle in the meniscal substance gives a fair indication of the stability of the meniscal rim. More than one meniscus must be felt before an accurate assessment can be made, but this should not be taken as a licence to poke needles into healthy menisci at will.

5. Synovial biopsy. Synovial biopsy in the suprapatellar pouch using forceps inserted through an instrument cannula from the lateral supratellar approach is simple and yields excellent specimens for histological study, as well as providing an opportunity to become familiar with the insertion of the cannula and handling of the instruments. The medial suprapatellar plica is a convenient structure for biopsy and can also be divided with operating scissors from this approach. Experience in handling the operating arthroscope can also be obtained at this stage by inserting the arthroscope from the antero-lateral route and manipulating the instruments in the supratellar pouch, but attempts at cutting menisci are unwise.

6. Probing hooks. The use of the jointline needle is helpful in developing the visuo-spacial co-ordination necessary for manipulating probing hooks inserted from the antero-medial approach, and synovial biopsy from the lateral suprapatellar approach provides experience in handling both cannula and instruments. The first antero-medial insertion of the instruments should be deferred until a patient is found who would otherwise require an antero-medial arthrotomy. Bucket handle tears of the medial meniscus are the commonest lesions of this sort and may be manipulated with a blunt hook passed along an instrument cannula (Fig. 6.9) placed just above the anterior horn of the medial meniscus and about 1 cm from the medial edge of the patellar tendon—a little lower and more medial than the ideal point of insertion for the excision of a meniscal fragment. Care should be taken not to prang the end of the arthroscope with the tip of the trocar as it is inserted by taking the precautions against this accident already described in Chapter 3.

Once inserted, the hook may be passed slowly, gently and under direct arthroscopic vision at all times to the medial meniscus, which may be picked up and manipulated as described in Chapter 2. When the medial meniscus can be manipulated easily, it is safe to try the higher and more lateral insertion needed for examination of the lateral meniscus. When fully confident in all aspects of the probing hook, and not a moment sooner, it is safe to excise simple meniscal lesions, but to attempt this before the probing hook can be manipulated easily and without damage to articular cartilage is foolhardy.

7. Removing flap and tags. Lesions suitable for the first arthroscopic procedure include excision of a stub of anterior cruciate ligament long enough to be caught between the joint surfaces and to cause mechanical symptoms (Fig. 5.22) and detached bucket handle fragments of medial meniscus (Fig. 6.17). Flaps arising from the under-surface of the meniscus are not suitable for excision at this stage. The probing hook will help to identify simple lesions which lie to the front of the joint and can easily be picked off with operating instruments.

When a suitable flap or tag has been found, it should be grasped firmly at its base with punch forceps or rongeurs, and removed. This type of lesion should not require trimming of the remaining rim and any attempt at such trimming is likely to cause more harm than good. Although removal of these lesions is quick, simple and satisfactory, the surgeon must still restrain himself from attacking large bucket-handle fragments or parrot-beak tears and must also be prepared to abandon the attempt and proceed to arthrotomy if difficulty is encountered.

8. Bucket handle tears. When the removal of flaps and tags at the front of the joint has become simple, the surgeon should look for a suitable bucket handle tear. The easiest bucket handle fragments with which to deal are those Type 1 tears of the medial meniscus that are less than 5 mm wide (Fig. 6.2), and the procedure will be less difficult if there is also a ruptured anterior cruciate ligament. Thicker fragments are more difficult and placement of the instruments must be precise if the intercondylar notch is occupied by a stout anterior cruciate ligament as well as a thick bucket handle fragment. The different techniques for excision have already been described in Chapter 4.

9. Complex meniscal tears. Having successfully dealt with a Type 1 bucket handle tear, it is safe to proceed to the management of Type 2 and Type 3 peripheral tears, thicker bucket handle fragments, and the pursuit of loose bodies, but it is wise to wait a little longer before tackling an extensive parrot beak tear or a thick posterior third tear of the medial meniscus. When these lesions can be dealt with simply, the surgeon will be able to direct his own progress and move on to other procedures.

Single puncture techniques

The single puncture technique is most easily learned with the simple biopsy forceps and narrow telescope supplied with some diagnostic arthroscopes, because the diagnostic telescope can be removed and replaced with operating instruments at any stage without waiting for a suitable case. The main difficulties likely to be encountered are those of poor visibility, already described in Chapter 3. Although practice in the suprapatellar pouch with the simple biopsy forceps or the operating arthroscope is possible as soon as the arthroscope can be handled confidently, the use of these instruments does not eliminate the need to learn the double puncture technique as well. An exception to this rule may be made for rheumatologists, whose main use for the arthroscope is the removal of synovial biopsy specimens from the supratellar pouch.

Aids to learning

Models of the knee are available for practising arthroscopy and arthroscopic surgery, but none is quite as good as the live human knee. The very realistic models made by True Models Corporation (Fig. 7.1) are excellent for practice in the basic skills of arthroscopy or arthroscopic surgery, and use of these models may both shorten the learning period and accelerate the development of the necessary visuo-spacial skills (Fig. 7.2).

As a teaching aid, the cadaver knee or amputation specimen is less satisfactory than a True Models knee. The inevitable mess associated with the use of any cadaveric specimen is increased in the case of arthroscopy by the need to distend the synovial cavity. The cell membranes lose their function after death so that distension of the knee with saline results in exudation of fluid from the joint and a large extra-articular collection of saline which tracks to the point of insertion of the instrument, where it leaks out and dribbles down the arthroscope to the trainee's hand,

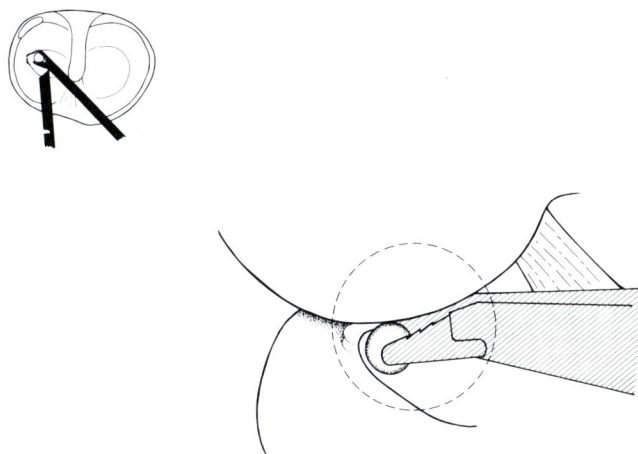

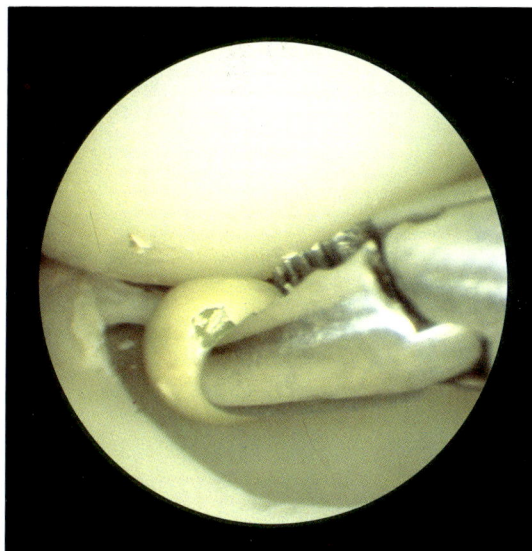

Fig. 7.1 Removing a dried pea from the lateral compartment of a True Models knee

elbow, and sometimes his eye. To add to these formidable difficulties, the cadaveric knee is stiff, whole leg amputation specimens are unwieldy and difficult to hold steady, and the view inside the cadaveric knee is quickly obscured by debris. For these reasons, arthroscopy is more difficult and less satisfactory in the cadaveric than in a live bleeding human knee or in a True Model.

A simple aid to develop the visuo-spacial skills may be made by placing a variety of everyday objects in a box and drilling holes, through which the arthroscope or probing instruments can be passed at various points

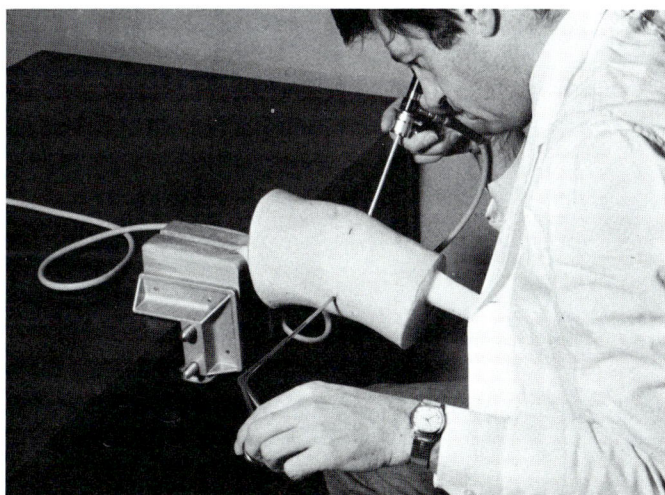

Fig. 7.2 Practising the manipulation of operating instruments inserted from the postero-medial approach using the True Models knee

in the wall of the box. These devices can offer nothing more than familiarity with the instruments and do not reproduce the cramped field of vision found within the knee, but they are cheap and easy to produce and their use can do no harm.

Dual viewing aids

Dual viewing teaching aids help to familiarise the novice with the view down the arthroscope and to ensure that trainees examine the knee correctly (Fig. 7.3). They also help to reduce the boredom of operating theatre staff, who have been known to tire of the uninterrupted view of the back of a surgeon's hat. Dual viewing aids may incorporate either a lens system to produce a true optical picture (Fig. 7.4), or a flexible fibre optic cable. Each system has its advantages and disadvantages and the selection of a teaching aid is a matter of individual choice dependent on many factors, of which one is likely to be the cost. Whatever the cost, the acquisition of a dual viewing aid will increase the acceptability of arthroscopy and arthroscopic surgery to colleagues and operating theatre staff, and is a sound investment.

Television

Provided that adequate funds are available, the dual viewing aid may be linked to a television camera and monitor, so that everyone within the operating theatre

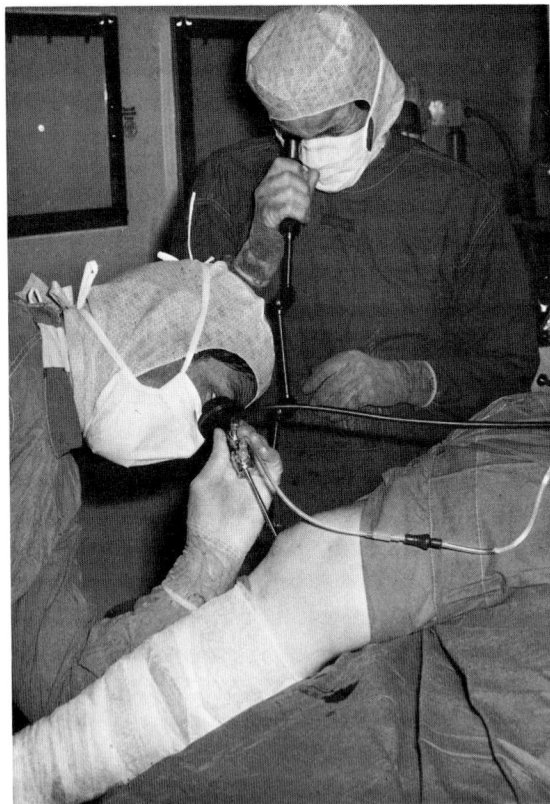

Fig. 7.3 The articulated dual viewing aid in use

can share the arthroscopic view. While this arrangement is excellent in theory, there are several difficulties in practice. The articulated optical link with the camera limits the mobility of the arthroscope making the examination more difficult, and the mobility of the link causes the picture to rotate alarmingly (Fig. 7.5). Unless the surgeon is able to operate the arthroscope and operating instruments while watching the television monitor instead of applying his eye to the arthroscope, correct orientation of the picture can only be achieved with the help of an assistant who can rotate the optical link synchronously with the arthroscope.

All these aids are helpful in shortening the learning period and in increasing the confidence of the surgeon. Even if none is available, the learning process can still be satisfactory for the surgeon and safe for the patient provided the surgeon only attempts procedures that he knows to be within his competence and observes the three basic rules of arthroscopic surgery which are:

1. Identify the pathology precisely
2. Always keep the tip of the operating instrument in view
3. Never cut blindly.

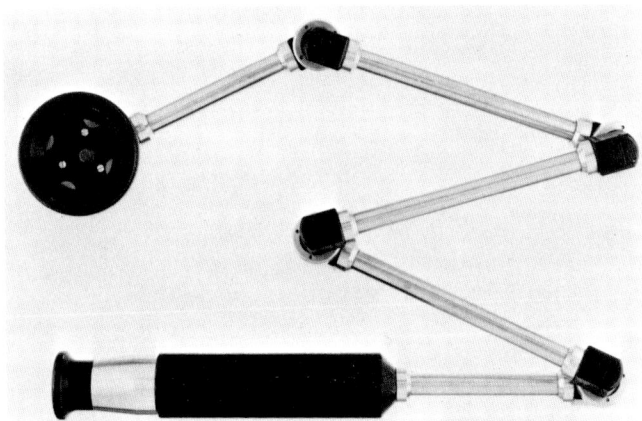

Fig. 7.4 The articulated dual viewing aid

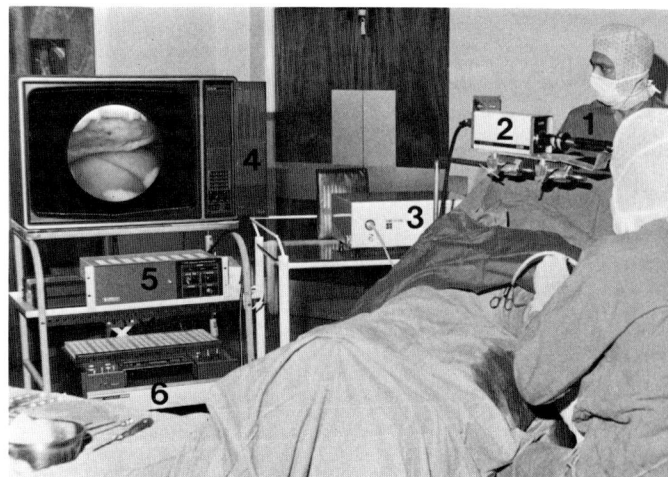

Fig. 7.5 Displaying the arthroscopic view on a television monitor (4). The arthroscope is connected by an articulated dual viewing aid (1) to a television camera (2). A high intensity light source (3) is required. (5) Camera control unit; (6) video-cassette recorder

8

Results and clinical experience

The introduction of any new surgical technique is bound to affect many aspects of clinical practice, including the bed occupancy, the demands on the physiotherapy department, the number of operations performed and the pattern of Out-Patient referrals. Before embarking on arthroscopic surgery of the knee, the surgeon will wish to know how his practice is likely to be affected and might, on reflection, choose to set the procedure aside and leave it to others.

Length of stay in hospital

Diagnostic arthroscopy can easily be performed as an out-patient 'day case' procedure, and most arthroscopic procedures can also be managed as day cases once the surgeon is adept. The advantages of day case surgery depend on many factors, among them the pressure on hospital beds, the facilities for out-patient surgery and the way in which health care is financed. It is also worth noting that the bed occupancy figures which loom so large in the minds of some hospital administrators in the United Kingdom are usually compiled on the basis of the number of beds occupied at midnight, and thus do not include patients who were discharged on the day of operation. The result of this is that a large number of out-patient procedures can have a disastrous effect on the hospital statistics when they depend more on the bed occupancy figure than on the number of patients treated.

When learning arthroscopic surgery, it is sensible to admit the patient on the day before the operation and to delay discharge until at least the day after. Patients should be advised that although it is very likely that they will be able to return home on the day after the operation, it may be necessary in certain circumstances to delay their discharge for several days. Patients should also be warned that however much effort is made to avoid opening their knee, this step may be necessary if the operation cannot be performed arthroscopically for any reason.

In practice, delay in discharge is exceptional. While the experience of all arthroscopic procedures is remarkably similar, the experience of meniscectomy offers a convenient yardstick with which to compare the arthroscopic and open techniques. Of the author's first 30 arthroscopic meniscectomies, 22 patients were able to return home on the day of operation or the day after, seven on the second day after operation, and one patient who had a cystic lateral meniscus on the fourth day. Of the second 30 patients, one stayed in hospital until the fourth day after operation because of a severe attack of migraine, and one stayed until the second day because of difficulties in arranging transport home. Since then, all patients have been able to return home within 24 hours of operation. For the nurses on the ward, this short stay in hospital results in an uneven distribution of work through the week, with peaks around the operating days and troughs at other times, including weekends. The overall bed occupancy of the ward also falls so that fewer beds are needed to achieve the same patient throughput, a matter of considerable economic importance.

Duration of operation

The length of the operation is its greatest disadvantage in the early stages. If a meniscus can be removed neatly and without fuss through a small arthrotomy in 15 minutes, there has to be a good reason for turning instead to an operation that may take almost two hours to perform and is attended by considerable frustration on the part of surgeon and operating theatre staff, who are unable to watch the operation or comprehend the surgeon's difficulties.

The reduction in the number of operations performed together with the reduction in the length of hospital admission can be demoralising for staff at all levels. Not surprisingly, tales of the length of operation tend to be exaggerated but the following figures should destroy the myth of the four-hour meniscectomy. Of the first 30 meniscectomies in the author's series, eight required more than one hour between the insertion of the irrigation needle in the suprapatellar pouch and the cutting of the last stitch. The mean operating time was 43 minutes, with a range of 10–90 minutes. During this period, three attempts at closed meniscectomy were abandoned and an open meniscectomy performed instead. Five of the second group of 30 closed meniscectomies took over an hour, with a mean operating time of 37 minutes and a range of 10–105 minutes, and no attempts at closed meniscectomy were abandoned. In the third group of 30 patients, three procedures took over one hour, the mean operating time was 34.5 minutes with a range of 12–75 minutes, and there were no abandoned procedures. It is now most unusual for a meniscectomy to take more than 50 minutes and the mean operating time has become steady at 22 minutes. Excision of a synovial shelf with the operating arthroscope or a lateral release take a very predictable 10–15 minutes from start to finish and other procedures, such as the removal of loose bodies, are variable in duration but rarely occupy more than 45 minutes. The operating time is prolonged by the taking of photographs, demonstrating to students and visitors or displaying the operation on television monitors, and the additional time spent in these pursuits has been disregarded in the operating times mentioned above.

When planning an operating list, it is helpful to know that four arthroscopic procedures can easily be accommodated in a three and a half hour operating session, and that this number may be increased to six if the cases include nothing more complicated than synovial biopsy, excision of a synovial shelf, lateral release, or a purely diagnostic arthroscopy.

Although further shortening of the operating time is likely with practice, the possibility of reducing the average duration of operating time much below 20 minutes seems unlikely. Nevertheless, the reduction of the operating time to a reliable 30 minutes makes out-patient arthroscopic meniscectomy an entirely acceptable and practical proposition.

Rehabilitation

The greatest single advantage of arthroscopic surgery is the dramatic reduction in the time required for return to work and normal everyday activities. Again using arthroscopic meniscectomy for comment, only one quarter of the first 60 patients needed physiotherapy after discharge and these 15 patients attended for an average of 5.1 treatments to make a total of 1.3 out-patient physiotherapy treatments after discharge for each patient in the whole group. Out-patient physiotherapy was usually required in patients whose knees had been locked for several weeks before operation, but gentle encouragement in full straight leg raising was also required in some patients with comparatively small tears. Ultrasound was sometimes applied to the two puncture wounds on either side of the patellar tendon, usually in top-class athletes anxious to cut every imaginable corner on the road to recovery.

The time taken for patients to return to work was also reduced, but varied according to the intra-articular pathology and the patient's occupation. Those patients engaged in light work were fit to return to their normal occupation after a mean of 5.9 days (range 2–27 days) and those engaged in heavy work after 14.1 days (range 6–40 days). The mean time taken for return to working fitness for the whole group was 9.6 days with a range of 2–40 days, but recovery was slower if the knee was affected by osteoarthrosis or a major ligament injury. The mean time for return to work in patients with no pathology apart from a meniscus lesion was 8.1 days, compared with 11.9 days for those with additional disorders. These results are comparable with those of Oretorp and Gillquist (1979).

One unforeseen difficulty in the achievement of early return to work in a welfare state is the understandable tendency of family practitioners unfamiliar with the technique to issue Certificates of Incapacity for six weeks on hearing that the patient has undergone a meniscectomy. In some circumstances the patient may be content with this decision if there is little or no incentive for him to request an early return to work, and may even consider it his right and privilege. This difficulty can be resolved by examining the patient in the out-patient clinic one week after discharge from hospital so that a certificate of fitness can be supplied.

Arthroscopic meniscectomy has sometimes attracted publicity because it enables athletes to return to sporting activities more quickly than journalists have come to expect. The return to full sporting fitness varies according to the individual and the sport concerned, but some patients have been able to return to competitive football within 10 days. Although the impact of arthroscopic surgery upon athletic injuries cannot be ignored, the early return to work of wage-earners and self-employed tradesmen is of greater importance.

Complications

Remarkably few complications have so far been described, but arthroscopic surgery is young, and it is inevitable that new complications will be reported in the future. The surgeon must therefore be intensely self critical, and should keep a careful record of his patients and their progress.

Broken instruments. The fracture of instruments within the knee is perhaps the greatest technical anxiety (Fig. 8.1). In the first 500 procedures, four such incidents occurred. In one, the tip of a small tenotomy blade introduced at the medial jointline fractured as a meniscal fragment was divided. The fragment of blade was so small and so firmly embedded in the medial ligament that the decision was made to leave the fragment rather than to proceed to an extensive dissection that would have been likely to result in more harm than good. Two years after this

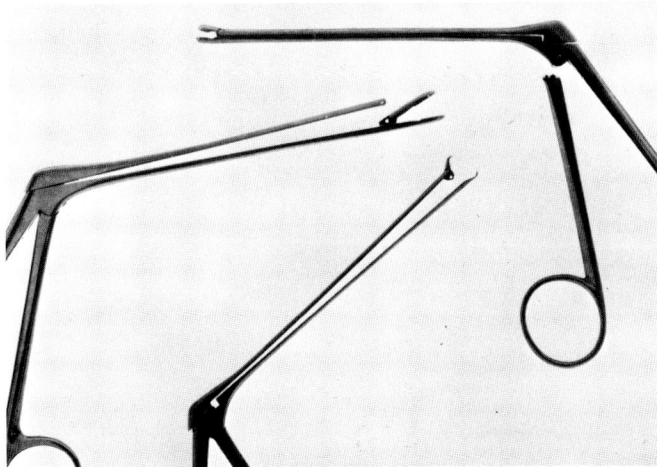

Fig. 8.1 These instruments broke during use but were withdrawn without leaving a fragment of metal in the knee

incident, the patient remains symptom free. The practice of inserting a tenotomy knife at the jointline was tried by the author in the early stages of developing the technique, but it did not prove helpful and is no longer recommended.

In a second patient, the tip of a percutaneous hypodermic needle used to manipulate a flap of lateral meniscus was severed with the punch forceps used to remove the meniscal fragment. The patient, an athlete, was particularly anxious to avoid an arthrotomy and successfully returned to competitive sport four days after operation. Subsequent radiographs showed the fragment localised in the soft tissues of the intercondylar notch.

A pair of prototype scissors fractured at a brazed joint as a synovial shelf was being divided by the double puncture technique. The distal end of the scissors separated and came to rest in the posterolateral compartment in such a way that the tips of the blades penetrated the posterior joint capsule with the other end of the instrument wedged firmly in the intercondylar notch. A small lateral arthrotomy was necessary to remove the fragment. In a fourth patient, a fragment of steel measuring 2 mm × 2 mm × 0.5 mm separated from the tip of a guillotine and was successfully retrieved without opening the joint. Fracture of the instruments is a real problem during the early stages, and great care must be exercised to prevent this complication by avoiding excessive loading or twisting of the instruments.

Synovial fistula. One early patient (the ninth arthroscopic meniscectomy) developed a clear watery discharge from the antero-medial wound on the ninth post-operative day and was considered to have a synovial fistula. The wound became dry after immobilisation in a plaster cylinder for seven days and the patient's recovery proceeded uneventfully thereafter. Although the presence of a synovial fistula was not proved conclusively, the diagnosis seems likely.

Deep vein thrombosis. To determine the exact incidence of deep vein thrombosis and other complications is difficult, but the experience of a group of surgeons who have together performed several thousand arthroscopic procedures suggests that the incidence of diagnosed deep vein thrombosis is in the region of one or two per thousand operations. While such evidence is little more than anecdotal, deep vein thrombosis does not appear to be an important practical problem, although it does occur occasionally.

Infection. The questionable sterility of arthroscopic surgery has already been mentioned and it is therefore reassuring to know that wound infection is almost unknown following arthroscopic procedures. Three or four infected haematomata following lateral release and one joint infection are known to have occurred around the world, representing a very approximate infection rate of 0.01 per cent. This low incidence is no excuse for carelessness, and every effort to avoid touching the tips of instruments entering the joint should be maintained at all times.

Effusion and haemarthrosis. In the author's experience, no haemarthroses have occurred and only one patient has developed an effusion requiring aspiration after operation. Effusion has not been a problem in patients who have deferred flexion until one week after operation, although some patients who began flexion of the knee during the first week after operation developed a moderate effusion that lasted for several weeks. If a persistent effusion develops, the patient should be advised to stop all sporting activities, to wear a crepe bandage around the knee to minimise the risk of the knee being flexed accidentally, and an inflammatory drug prescribed. Some surgeons have encountered an incidence of troublesome effusion in the region of 2–6 per cent, while others report none at all. The reason for this discrepancy is not apparent.

Wound tenderness. A little thickening and tenderness is common around either wound, although the medial wound is more often affected than the lateral. This thickening, which is presumably due to

a small haematoma, is seldom troublesome and can be expected to settle within three weeks of operation.

Articular cartilage damage. Scuffing of the articular cartilage becomes less common with experience, but is difficult to avoid completely (Fig. 8.2). The irregularity, however slight, is magnified by the arthroscope and it is comforting to know that the apparent defects may prove impossible to find at arthrotomy. No ill-effect has been observed from this minor intra-articular cartilage damage and repeat arthroscopic examination a few months later suggests that it heals well, but care must be taken nevertheless to minimise trauma to the articular cartilage during operation.

Medico-legal complications. Medico-legal considerations are of more importance in some parts of the world than others. Anxieties about the fracture of instruments within the knee and reoperation for persistent symptoms are well founded, and a particular source of anxiety is the surgeon who attempts arthroscopic surgery before he is properly competent at arthroscopy. It is a matter of professional responsibility for a surgeon to attempt only those procedures within his competence, as outlined in the previous chapter. To embark on arthroscopic surgery after purchasing a set of powered instruments and an operating arthroscope is a recipe for disaster that can only bring the individual surgeon, and arthroscopic surgery in general, into disrepute.

A further source of anxiety is the patient who has

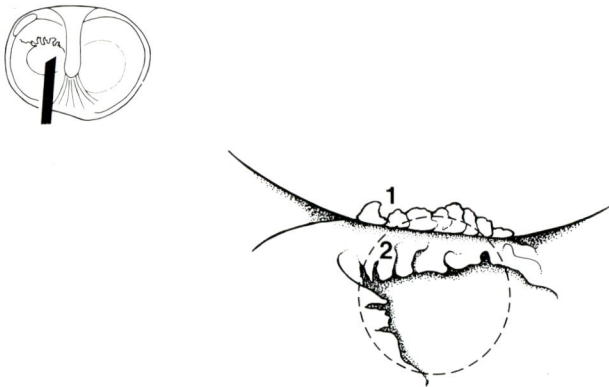

Fig. 8.2 Damage to the under-surface of the lateral femoral condyle (1) caused by attempts to trim the lateral meniscus (2) with cutting instruments passed directly across the joint space between the tibial plateau and femoral condyle

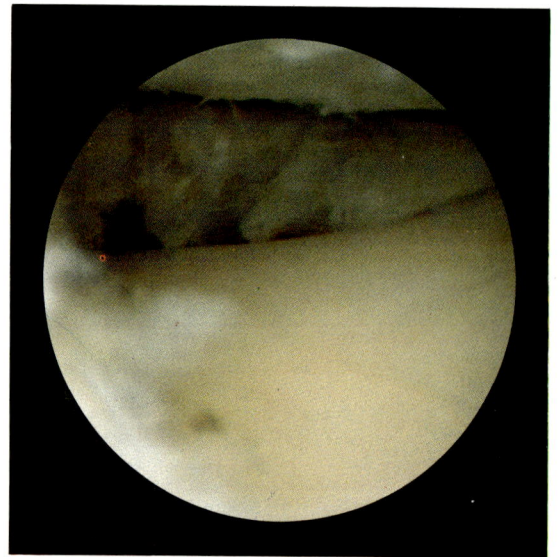

a poor prognosis and expects miracles. However skilled the arthroscopist may be, any knee with degenerative change or a major ligament injury has a poor outlook and the surgeon should protect himself by explaining this to the patient in the plainest possible language as well as recording his opinion in his own records and in the letter to the patient's general practitioner.

It is comforting to know that in the fullness of time, when arthroscopy has become the rule rather than the exception, the position of a surgeon who operates upon a knee without being able to perform an arthroscopy is likely to be indefensible, but until that day comes any surgeon who practises arthroscopic surgery is strongly advised to guard his rear and practise defensive medicine.

Pattern of referral

The surgeon who takes up arthroscopic surgery of the knee must expect to suffer an alteration in the pattern of his work. The difference between the results of arthroscopic and open surgery of the knee is so striking that patients with disorders of the knee quickly come to dominate the practice of any surgeon who offers this technique and, while few would consciously seek to be a 'one operation' surgeon, such a fate may be difficult to avoid.

Although the results of arthroscopic surgery are remarkably successful, the procedures themselves are technically exacting, often frustrating, and the character of the operations is so different from the rest of orthopaedic surgery that many surgeons may well find them uncongenial. To give up a technique as successful as arthroscopic surgery is difficult, and it might be very reasonable to decide, in retrospect, that it would have been better not to have become involved and to have left this type of surgery to others.

Looking to the future, it is possible to imagine the time when orthopaedic surgery will be sub-divided in much the same way as 'general' surgery has now become. Hand surgery, joint replacement surgery, scoliosis surgery, spinal surgery and childrens' orthopaedics are ready candidates for such specialisation. The introduction of a new surgical technique that is both difficult to learn and highly successful may well provide an impetus for the development of knee surgery as another speciality within the orthopaedic family. Whether such development is for good or ill is for the reader to consider, and the future to decide.

REFERENCE

Oretorp N, Gillquist J 1979 Transcutaneous Meniscectomy under Arthroscopic Control. International Orthopaedics 3:19–25

Index